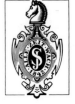

F. Hadžiselimović

Cryptorchidism

Management and Implications

With Contributions by
W.J. Cromie F. Hinman B. Höcht S.J. Kogan
T.S. Trulock J.R. Woodard

Foreword by F. Hinman

With 67 Figures

Springer-Verlag
Berlin Heidelberg NewYork 1983

Privatdozent Dr. Faruk Hadžiselimović
Basler Kinderspital
Römergasse 8
CH-4005 Basel

For explanation of the cover motive see legend to Fig. 8, p. 23.

ISBN 3-540-11881-0 Springer-Verlag Berlin Heidelberg New York
ISBN 0-387-11881-0 Springer-Verlag New York Heidelberg Berlin

Library of Congress Cataloging in Publication Data. Hadžiselimović, Faruk, 1944-. Cryptorchidism, management and implications. 1. Cryptorchidism. I. Cromie, W.J. (William, J.), 1943-. II. Title. RJ477.5.C74H33 1983 616.6'8 82-19184 ISBN 0-387-11881-0 (U.S.).

Reproduction of figures: Gustav Dreher GmbH, Stuttgart

Typesetting, printing and bookbinding: Universitätsdruckerei H. Stürtz AG, Würzburg

2122/3130-543210

Contributors

Cromie, W.J., Professor Dr., The Albany Medical College of Union University, Albany, N.Y. 12208/USA

Hinman, F., Jr., Professor Dr., Department of Urology, University of San Francisco, San Francisco, California/USA

Höcht, B., Privatdozent Dr., University Hospital Würzburg, Department of Children Surgery, D-8700 Würzburg

Kogan, S.J., Professor Dr., Division of Pediatric Urology and Pediatric Renal Transplantation, Albert Einstein College of Medicine and Montefiore Hospital and Medical Center, Bronx, N.Y./USA

Trulock, T.S., Dr., Emory University, Atlanta, Georgia/USA

Woodard, J.R., Professor Dr., Emory University School of Medicine, Chief of Urology at the Henrietta Egleston Hospital for Children, Atlanta, Georgia/USA

To Ellen
– my wife and the mother
of our 4 children

Acknowledgments

It is my great pleasure to thank my colleagues at the University Children's Hospital in Basle and all those who, directly or indirectly, have helped to bring this book into being.

The idea of developing the book was formed by F. Hinman Jr. during two symposia on undescended testes held in Detroit (October 1980) and in Boston (May 1981).

I am very grateful to Prof. G. Stalder for his constant encouragement and constructive criticism. Special thanks is due to those colleagues whose written contributions enhance the book, and I am indebted to Dr. U. Bühler and Dr. M. von der Ohe for their advice and help. Also, I am thankful to the Swiss National Foundation, Höchst AG, and the Swiss Cancer League, who through their financial support made this work possible. I wish to thank my friend Tim McCarthy sincerely for the translation. Lastly, I would like to express my gratitude to Mrs. N. Proschek for countless hours of patient work in typing and retyping the manuscript.

F. Hadžiselimović

Foreword

Ferment, a sign of progress in any scientific field, has previously been lacking in the area of cryptorchidism, where the only activity has been in improving operative methods. Now, however, profound changes in the care of boys with cryptorchidism are being brought about; ideas are arising from a fresh look at comparative anatomy, and histological and experimental observations are being supplemented by clinical tests made possible by new hormonal agents.

The treatment of cryptorchidism begins with its recognition by the pediatrician, who until now has shown little interest because of disappointing results from chorionic gonadotropin administration. As for the surgeon, his bent toward restoration of normal anatomical relationships has kept his attention focused on the development of better surgical technics to bring the recalcitrant testis into the scrotum. Both specialists have avoided the primordial question of why the testis did not descend properly. If this were known they would treat the cause of cryptorchidism, and not be satisfied merely with trying to correct its end result.

As one reads this book, one sees that in most patients cryptorchidism is not caused by some anatomical structure blocking the way or by some deformity of the testis interfering with the transport mechanism. Rather, deficiencies in the hormonal environment of the fetus retard the developmental sequences essential to the normal differentiation and descent of the testis. The clinical solution is thus to provide the deficient substances.

Careful investigation of the embryogenesis of the normal and the cryptorchid fetus, combined with critical experiments on hormonal manipulation in animals, has led Dr. Hadžiselimović to a rational method of treatment, made clinically possible by the concurrent development of the essential hormonal substance. His findings are then related to current concepts of infertility, malignancy, and surgical therapy.

Clearly, the reader of this book will be led into the modern era of cryptorchidism therapy.

San Francisco   F. Hinman

Contents

1 Introduction
F. Hadžiselimović   1

2 History and Evolution of Testicular Descent
F. Hadžiselimović (with 3 Figures)   3
  2.1 History of Research into Testicular Descent and Maldescent   3
  2.2 Evolution of Testicular Descent   6
References   8

Implications

3 Embryology of Testicular Descent and Maldescent
F. Hadžiselimović (with 17 Figures) 11
  3.1 Indifferent Stage of Gonadal Development 11
  3.2 Differentiation of the Testis 12
    3.2.1 Germ Cells 12
    3.2.2 Sertoli Cells 15
    3.2.3 Leydig Cells 15
  3.3 Male Duct Differentiation and Development 17
    3.3.1 Development of the Testis Coverings 21
    3.3.2 Comparison of Testicular Descent in Humans and
        Rodents 23
  3.4 Estrogen-Induced Cryptorchidism 25
  3.5 Spondaneous Congenital Cryptorchidism in Mice:
    Treatment with GnRH 26
  3.6 Morphology and Histology of the Cryptorchid Epididymis 28
References 33

4 Histology and Ultrastructure of Normal and Cryptorchid Testes
F. Hadžiselimović (with 18 Figures) 35
  4.1 Development of the Normal Testis in Children 35
    4.1.1 First Year of Life 35
    4.1.2 Fourth Year 35
    4.1.3 Puberty 35
  4.2 Development of the Cryptorchid Testis 45
    4.2.1 Behavior of the Number of Spermatogonia in Cryptor-
        chid Gonads 45
        4.2.1.1 In Relation to Age 45
        4.2.1.2 In Relation to Position 47
    4.2.2 Ultrastructure of Cryptorchid Testis 48
        4.2.2.1 Germ Cells 48
        4.2.2.2 Sertoli Cells 50

         4.2.2.3 Peritubular Connective Tissue 50
         4.2.2.4 Leydig Cells 52
    4.2.3 Congenital or Acquired Lesions? Iatrogenic
         Cryptorchidism 53
    4.2.4 Frequency and Ultrastructure of Carcinoma In Situ
         Cells in the Testes of Cryptorchid Children 55
  References 58

5 Endocrinology of the Hypothalamo-Pituitary-Gonadal Axis
  F. Hadžiselimović (with 5 Figures) 59
  5.1 Development of the Hypothalamo-Pituitary-Gonadal Axis
     During Intrauterine Life in Normal Males 59
  5.2 Development of the Hypothalamo-Pituitary-Gonadal Axis in
     Normal Boys 59
  5.3 Role of Leydig Cells 61
  5.4 Mechanism of Androgen Action 62
  5.5 Role of Sertoli Cells 64
  5.6 Testing of the Hypothalamo-Pituitary-Gonadal Axis Utilizing
     GnRH 64
  5.7 Development of the Hypothalamo-Pituitary-Gonadal Axis in
     Cryptorchid Boys 65
  References 68

6 Fertility in Cryptorchidism
  S.J. Kogan (with 5 Figures) 71
  6.1 Introduction 71
  6.2 Factors Influencing the Interpretation of Infertility Data in
     Cryptorchid Patients 71
    6.2.1 Patient Source 71
    6.2.2 Age at Treatment 71
    6.2.3 Medical VS Surgical Treatment 72
    6.2.4 Location of Testis 72
    6.2.5 Injury from Surgery 72
    6.2.6 Method of Sperm Analysis 72
    6.2.7 Definition of Infertility 72
  6.3 Analysis of Extant Fertility Data 73
  6.4 Special Considerations Regarding Fertility in Cryptoridism 73
  6.5 Correlation of HCG-Induced Descent and Subsequent Fertility 73
  6.6 Fertility in Cryptorchid Patients with Compensatory Testicular
     Hypertrophy 74
  6.7 Evidence for a Contralateral Lesion in the Descended Testis 75
  References 81

7 Cryptorchidism and Malignant Testicular Disease
  W.J. Cromie (with 3 Figures) 83
  7.1 Etiologic Theories of Malignant Degeneration 83
  7.2 General Risk Factors in Testicular Cancer 83
  7.3 Premalignant Histologic Changes in the Cryptorchid Gonad 86
  7.4 Tumor Cell Types in Undescended Testes 87
  7.5 Incidence and Risk Analysis of Malignant Disease with Crypt-
     orchidism 88
  7.6 Theoretical Considerations 90
  References 91

Treatment

8   Examinations and Clinical Findings in Cryptorchid Boys
     F. Hadžiselimović (with 1 Figure)   93
     8.1 Incidence 93
     8.2 Position and Side Affected   93
     8.3 Concomitant Findings   94
          8.3.1 Mental and Somatic Retardation   94
          8.3.2 Heredity   94
          8.3.3 Torsion of Testis 95
          8.3.4 Hernias, Renal Failure, and Genital Malformations 95
          8.3.5 Psychic Alterations 95
     8.4 Examination Technique   95
     References   98

9   Indications and Contraindications for Orchiopexy
     F. Hinman, Jr.   99
     9.1 Perform Orchiopexy   99
     9.2 Perform Orchiectomy   99
     9.3 Omit Surgical Treatment   99
     References 100

10   Hormonal Treatment
     F. Hadžiselimović (with 9 Figures) 101
     10.1 HCG Treatment   101
     10.2 GnRH Treatment   101
     References 114

11   Surgical Treatment of Cryptorchidism
     J.R. Woodard and T.S. Trulock (with 5 Figures) 115
     11.1 Introduction   115
     11.2 Preoperative Localization of the Testis 115
     11.3 Surgical Techniques 116
          11.3.1 Standard Orchiopexy 116
          11.3.2 Staged Orchiopexy 117
          11.3.3 Fowler-Stephens (Long-Loop Vas) Orchiopexy . .   120
          11.3.4 Microsurgical (Autotransplantation) Technique . 122
          11.3.5 Neonatal Transabdominal Orchiopexy   124
     References 125

12   Conclusions
     F. Hadžiselimović   127
     12.1 The Role of the Epididymis in Testicular Descent 127
     12.2 Clinical and Pathophysiological Implications in Cryptorchid
          Boys   127

13   Treatment Schedule
     F. Hadžiselimović   129

14   Prospectives
     F. Hadžiselimović and B. Höcht (with 1 Figure) 131
     References 132

Subject Index 133

1 Introduction

F. Hadžiselimović

To deal with cryptorchidism requires an understanding of the evolution of testicular descent, comparative anatomy, embryology, histology, ultrastructure, endocrinology, and particularly the clinical aspects of hormonal and surgical treatment. It is impossible to comprehend cryptorchidism purely from the viewpoint of endocrinology or pathology.

During the past 10 years significant progress has been made in all of these disciplines. Due to these advances, intrauterine hormonal dysfunction as a primary cause of cryptorchidism began to be revealed. There is little doubt today that in many cases testicular maldescent is due to impairment of the intrauterine hypothalamopituitary-gonadal axis. Consequently, hormonal therapy is progressively replacing surgery as the treatment of first choice. Until 1975, human chorionic gonadotropin (HCG) treatment was universally recommended. With the newly developed gonadotropin-releasing hormone (GnRH) nasal spray, a logical and effective medication, positive results have been achieved in randomized double-blind and other appropriate clinical trials.

In the early 1950s it was believed that the optimal time to treat cryptorchidism was at puberty, based on the histological findings of the day from Charny and Wolgin. In their opinion cryptorchid testes were congenitally damaged, and surgery was performed mainly for cosmetic reasons. That the sterility rate in males with bilateral cryptorchidism was over 90% and in those with unilateral cryptorchidism was about 60% was believed to be congenitally predetermined. Numerous histological studies within the past 15 years have shown that there is continuous testicular development throughout childhood. After the 2nd year of life, the undescended testes develop an irreversible damage to their germ cells.

The old statement of Cooper (1925) claiming that the testes in cryptorchid infants closely resemble normal testes was recently proven. Over 80% of adults operated on for cryptorchidism during infancy were found to be fertile.

In this book an attempt has been made to explain the pathophysiological background of the development of cryptorchidism and to give a rational explanation for GnRH treatment. Other modern findings in the embryology of testicular descent in humans and rodents shed new light on the role of the epididymis. The improved methods of tissue preparation, as well as the ultrastructural examination of 721 biopsies of cryptorchid boys, showed that gonadotropin deficiency is the cause of undescended testes in at least three-quarters of all cases. This is especially evident when the ultrastructural findings (the status of the Leydig cells and the stage of germ cell development) are compared to the endocrinological results. The risk of developing testicular malignancy is significantly higher in cryptorchid males, a problem that is reexamined in this book. Also, the fertility rate, the indications, and the surgical approach are extensively described.

We hope that the book will be useful to practicing pediatricians and pediatric urologists, who can obtain herein an understanding of the etiology of cryptorchidism as well as the rationale and schedule for its treatment.

2 History and Evolution of Testicular Descent

F. Hadžiselimović

2.1 History of Research into Testicular Descent and Maldescent

The history of testicular descent is closely connected with the expression of masculinity and as such can be traced back to ancient Egypt. The eunuchs with their habitus were a well-described phenomenon. During the Middle Ages one of the precepts of canon law required that all candidates for the priesthood must have "duo testes bene pendulam" [1].

Research into testicular descent was initiated with Haller and Hunter [2, 3] (Figs. 1, 2). It was Hunter who discovered that the testes descend during embryonal life from the dorsal abdominal wall into the scrotum [3]. He was also the first to describe the gubernaculum as a governor of testicular descent.

The nineteenth century was a very interesting period for research into testicular descent, a time when intensive investigations of morphology and comparative anatomy were made. The much-admired works of Klaatsch and Frankel [4, 5] resulted from these investigations. Based on his observations of rodents, Klaatsch proposed the conus inguinalis as the key mechanism in testicular descent [4]. Active traction of the gubernaculum by its muscle power was unfortunately misinterpreted by Seiler in 1817 [6]. However, the active muscle traction theory of the gubernaculum or conus inguinalis was even at that time not generally accepted [7]. Around 1884, a group of investigators, strongly influenced by the works of Weil [7], denied that the gubernaculum had any active role in testicular descent. In their view, testicular descent was accomplished mainly by increased intra-abdominal pressure [7]. In 1847 Weber developed a "balloon" theory of the gubernaculum [8]. He hypothesized that a balloon-like swelling of the gubernaculum, presumably the musculus cremaster, is the main force for testicular descent [8]. This theory soon fell into oblivion because of the inability to prove by histology the existence of swelling of the cremaster during testicular descent.

Intensive research into this puzzling phenomenon was undertaken at the beginning of the twentieth century. It is peculiar that much less attention has been paid to the *why* of testicular descent than to the intense scrutiny of *how* testicular descent takes place. In 1900 Neuhauser [9] argued that the scrotum is a sexual signal to the female of capability to produce offspring. The German neurologist Müller contended that the existence of the scrotum is an art of self-creativity in a male body [10]. Commenting in

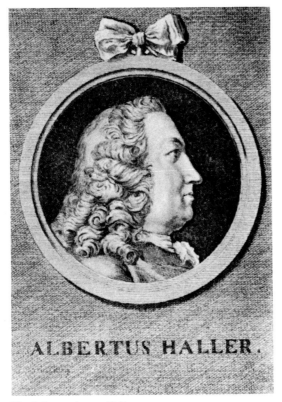

Fig. 1. Baron A. von Haller

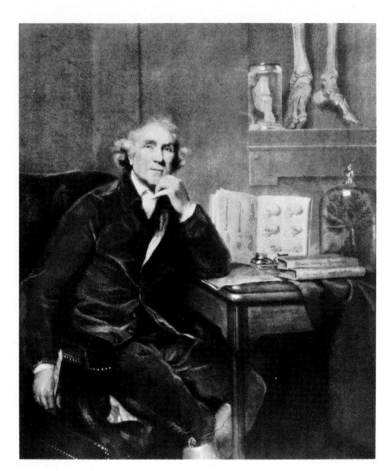

Fig. 2. John Hunter

the same book, Portmann [11] unfolded the *Gestaltungstheorie* or form theory. According to him, the expression of male sex constitutes self-creativity in the male body irrespective of any evolutionary reasons or the need of the testis to descend to a cooler region.

The thermoregulatory theory was based on experiments by Moore and his co-workers [12]. Having induced experimental cryptorchidism by surgically transferring the testis from the scrotum to the abdomen, just as Piana had done in 1891 [13], they observed degeneration of the intratubular epithelium identical with that of congenital cryptorchidism [12]. Their hypothesis that the human testis descends because of temperature factors is widely accepted. The main reservation with this theory is that it fails to explain why spermatogenesis is unimpaired in mammals bearing their testes intraabdominally during their whole life. The secondary adaptation of the gonads to a lower temperature is the most logical explanation.

In the early 1930s the first histological observation of the development of the normal testis and description of the cryptorchid testis were undertaken. It was undisputed that cryptorchid males were frequently sterile, and the belief of Hunter that the cryptorchid gonad does not descend because of dysgenesis was universally accepted. Cooper [13] was the first to criticize this theory. In her observations, the cryptorchid testes in very young children were histologically normal and the higher they were positioned the more expressed were the pathological changes [14]. It took nearly 50 years for this observation to be accepted.

In 1938 Moscowitsch asserted that cryptorchidism is an intersex state [15]. In his opinion the ligamentum posterior vesicale was primarily responsible for the failure in testicular descent.

In the same year, the first hormonal treatment of cryptorchidism was inaugurated [16]. This was the outcome of observing that hypophysectomy in rodents prevented testicular de-

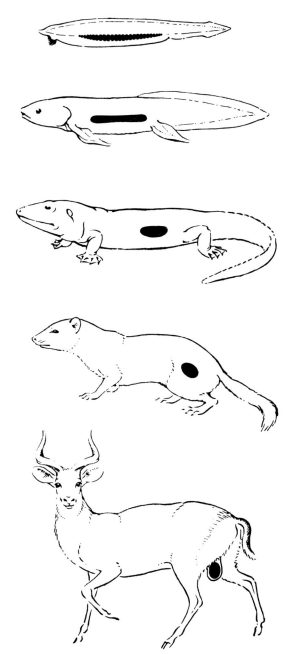

Fig. 3. Portmann's form theory. (Portmann A. [29])

therapy and others, particularly surgeons, stated that only retractile and not true cryptorchid testes responded to the treatment. There have always been attempts to prove definitively the key role of the gubernaculum in testicular descent and its function. The irritating point is that even with the absence or severance of the gubernaculum, testicular descent still takes place [18, 19].

In the past 15 years, irrespective of these observations, the old theories were described de novo and adapted, always promoting the gubernaculum as having the crucial role. Three recently developed theories give the gubernaculum this role:

1. Wensing [20] described the gubernaculum swelling as being a motor of testicular descent. This swelling should be independent of androgene and under the so-called factor X control. The main criticism of this theory is that if the testis is removed and its tissue replaced by a paraffin ball, descent occurs following the administration of androgenes [21, 22]. This was published for the first time in 1943 by Martins [21] and confirmed in recent experiments by Backhouse [22]. The experiments support the theory that the testicular mass is moved along the inguinal canal by a mechanism which is totally independent of other testicular factors except androgenes.

2. In 1981 Elder and co-workers described that a meander-shaped gubernaculum under dihydrotestosterone influence had induced testicular descent in rabbits [23]. They attempted to apply this concept universally to all mammals, even man. This explanation will hardly be universally accepted because in man there is no meander-shaped gubernaculum and because even if the gubernaculum is missing (regressed after birth) testicular descent does occur following hormonal treatment (see Chap. 10).

3. Between 1979 and 1981, when attention was focused on the musculus cremaster, serious endeavors were made to explain that the development of the processus vaginalis and the growth of the musculus cremaster under androgene influence were responsible for testicular descent [22]. It should be apparent from this study that testicular descent in man is not associated with any contractile forces by a classical fibromuscular guberna-

scent and the application of water-soluble extracts of the anterior pituitary induced testicular descent in these animals [17]. The initial results of hormonal therapy were promising, but very soon the failure of hormonal treatment to induce testicular descent and preserve fertility in numerous cases led to a division of opinion. Those on one side promoted HCG

culum traction [22]. Instead there is maintenance of a primitive mesenchymatous core in the inguinal and scrotal regions, which is not encroached upon by the developing body and scrotal wall structure [22]. The processus vaginalis must be adequately developed, as a prerequisite of testicular descent [22]. However, it appears uncommon to find a deficiency in the growth of the processus vaginalis and cremaster muscle as the only feature of the cryptorchid state unless there is a mechanical barrier to their development [22].

Weil's old hypothesis [7] of intra-abdominal pressure was again popular in the period from 1969 to 1975 [24]. Further to this concept, it was stated that a late closure in the weak triangle resulted in cryptorchidism [24]. As with all theories about the key role of the gubernaculum, this argument fails to explain why hormonal treatment in childhood (when neither the gubernaculum nor the weak triangle exist) induced descent. And finally, the theory of pelvic rotation and development as the main cause of testicular descent is generally unacceptable, because there are numerous testicond animals having pelvic rotation but completely lacking any testicular dislocation.

Based on the experimental replacement of the already-descended testis in its original position, an overwhelming number of researchers have attempted to explain the etiology of cryptorchidism. These studies make it abundantly clear how secondary testicular changes develop, but completely fail to explain the real pathophysiological background of cryptorchidism.

The malformation of the inguinal canal, causing a mechanical barrier to descent, is thought to be a frequent etiological factor in the development of cryptorchidism. In our clinical studies we found the mechanical barrier in only 3% of the patients operated on for cryptorchidism.

2.2 Evolution of Testicular Descent

Testicular descent, a process in which the gonad descends from the dorsal abdominal wall into the scrotum, occurs only within the mammalian species. Although the general opinion is that the process develops similarly in most mammals, the etiology of this puzzling procedure is still controversial and to a great extent unknown. No biological explanation of testicular descent has yet been found, but all those engaged in studying the etiology of human testicular descent come sooner or later to Portmann's form theory [11]. This theory maintains that mammals with completed descent are those in whom the head and anal poles have reached their highest development, in contrast to primitive and archaic mammals who show no differentiation of the anal and frontal poles, in whom testicular descent does not occur. The gonads appear as an organ which forms externally on mammals and expresses the male sex in a new manner (Fig. 3).

It would appear from comparative anatomical and experimental studies that the descent into the scrotum has been influenced primarily by the necessity of migration of the cauda epididymidis to the scrotal region [25]. Testicular descent is seen as a purely mechanical event, which enables the cauda epididymis to project from the body but has no significance for the biological function of the testis as such [25]. It should be stressed that the scrotum, and thus testicular descent, is a typical feature among mammals (Table 1). It is not only found in Euteria but is also common among Marsupials, indicating that it is a parallel development in the evolutionary process. One of the peculiarities is that only mammals living on the ground may have a scrotum. However, with regard to the evolution of mammals, it is possible to distinguish that the scrotum and thus descent is common in the evolutionarily younger species having also a differentiated stature. Within all recent mammalian orders we can observe mammals without testicular descent, those with incomplete descent, and finally a group where the descent is complete (Table 1). Even within each mammalian species all three forms of descent are evident. As a rule, it can be said that mammals which are naturally cryptorchid are also an evolutionarily older species. Androgen metabolism is probably an invariant feature of the Chordata and must be considered as an evolutionary advantage because it provides a subtle mechanism whereby a single hormonal stimulus, the parent androgen, may be modulated to elicit a varied spectrum of responses [26]. The androgens have a crucial role in testicular descent. In Monotremata there is no testicular

Table 1. Arrangement of mammalian species according to the type of epididymal descent. The numerical arrangement of species in parentheses is in accordance with [30]

	Cryptorchid (testicond)	Partial descensus	Descensus
Monotremata [1]	All		
Marsupialia [2]	Notoricidae	Vombatidae	Macropodidae
Hyracoidea [10]	Procaviidae		
Proboscidea [11]	Elephantidae		
Sirenia [12]	Trichechidae Dugongidae		
Insectivora [3]	Macroscelidae Chrysochloridae	Soricidae Tenrecidae	
Edentata [14]	Bradypodidae Myrmecophagidae	Dasypodidae	
Perissodactyla [8]		Rhinocerotidae Tapiridae	Equidae
Cetacea [13]		Delphinidae Physeteridae Balaenopteridae	
Tubulidentata [15]		Orycteropodidae	
Pholidota [16]		Manidae	
Rodentia [17]		Chinchillidae	Scuridae Muridae
Lagomorpha [18]			Leporidae
Chiroptera [5]			Phyllostomatidae
Dermoptera [4]			Cynocephalidae
Carnivora [7]		Phocidae	Canidae Ursidae Hyaenidae
Artiodactyla [9]		Hippopotamidae	Bovidae Camelidae Cervidae Giraffidae
Primates [6]		Lorisidae	Tupaiide Lemuridae Galagidae Cebidae Cercopithecidae Hylobatidae Pongidae Hominidae

descent, while in Marsupialia all three types of descent occur. Among Euteria, Insectivora are naturally cryptorchid although Soricidae have a partial descent. Edentata, Pholidata, and Cetacea are similar to Insectivora. In some families of Chiroptera, Dermoptera, Rodentia, Lagomorpha, and Carnivora and in most Ungu-lata and Primata complete testicular descent is evident. From the embryological point of view, the testes in Ruminantia and Primata are descended completely at birth and have the best-developed scrotum compared with other mammals. The transient stage is, in most mammals, characterized by descent of the epididymis while the testis remains in the inguinal region or intra-abdominally.

Darwin [27] comprehended that sexually dimorphic species are wont to have polygamous matings whereas the monomorphic ones are inclined to be a monogamous species. The large body size that distinguishes many long-living mammalian species is constantly linked with long gestation periods and a small litter, frequently only one offspring [27]. Thus the reproductive extent of a population is regulated by the number of breeding females it contains. A population cannot allow a reduction in the sum of these invaluable females by exposing them to too severe a selective influence [27]. Furthermore, since she produces so few descendants in her lifetime, the measure of genetic bestowal any one female contributes to the next generation of a population is easily gauged [27, 28].

With a polygamous way of life large mammalian species can compensate for a long gestation period as well as for long generation time and small litter size [27, 28].

Not extraordinarily, many of the large mammals are said to indulge in polygamous mating of the polygynous (many females) type, and with these species, Darwin was correct in coupling expressed sexual dimorphism with polygamy [27]. To enable this state of reproduction, the mammals have to possess the potential for repeated ejaculation. This is only achieved if the epididymis is lying in a cooler region to store the sperm. For this reason the descent of the epididymis and not the testis should be the evolutionary prerequisite for the polygynous way of life [25].

There is little question that the display of sexual dimorphism and the subsequent customs of polygynous mating were conducive to the extraordinary evolutionary success of mammals. Despite being sexually very dimorphic, our own species obviously owes its evolutionary prosperity, based on remarkable aptitude, to the practise of monogamy [27, 28]. Although polygyny has apparently been rare in human history, the proneness to it seems always to have been there; note the inclusion of such words as "harem" and "seraglio", in human vocabularies [28].

It would appear that a change from the polygynous to the monogamous mating system was attained by human ancestors without genetically decreasing the male's penchant toward skirmishing and polygamy [28]. Probably because of the sexual demarcation of labor noted above, a change from the polygynous to the monogamous mating system was achieved, not by eliminating preoccurring sexual dimorphism, but rather by adding specific female postpubertal developments to greatly increase sexual dimorphism [28].

References

1. Kleinteich B, Hadžiselimović F, Hesse V, Schreiber G (1979) Kongenitale Hodendystopien. VEB, Georg Thieme, Leipzig
2. Haller A von (1749) Hernie congenital. Goethingoe
3. Palmer JF (1837) The works of John Hunter, vol IV. Longman & Co., London
4. Klaatsch H (1890) Über den Descensus testiculorum. Morphol Jahrb 16:587–646
5. Frankl O (1900) Beiträge zur Lehre vom Descensus testiculorum. Sitzungsbuch der Akademie der Wissenschaften, Wien, Math. Nat. Cl., Abt. III:107–264
6. Seiler BW (1817) Observationes normalles de testiculorum ex abdomine in scrotum et partium genitalium anomaliis. Leipzig
7. Weil C (1884) Ueber den Descensus testiculorum. Prag
8. Weber EH (1847) Ueber den Descensus testiculorum beim Menschen und einigen Säugetieren. Müllers Archiv
9. Neuhauser, cit. from Müller A (1938) Individualität und Fortpflanzung als Polaritätserscheinung. Gustav Fischer, Jena, p 5
10. Müller A (1938) Individualität und Fortpflanzung als Polaritätserscheinung. Gustav Fischer, Jena
11. Portmann A (1938) Nachwort in: Individualität und Fortpflanzung als Polaritätserscheinung. Müller A (ed) Gustav Fischer, Jena, pp 59–63
12. Moore CR (1924) Properties of the gonads as controllers of somatic and psychical characteristics. Am J Anat 34:269–316
13. Cooper ERA (1929) The histology of the retained testis in the human subject at different ages and its comparison with the scrotal testis. J Anat 64:5–27
14. Southam AH, Cooper ERA (1927) Hunterian lecture on the pathology and treatment of the retained testis in childhood. Lancet 1:805–811
15. Moskowicz L (1934) Die Entstehung des Kryptorchismus. Arch f klin Chir 179:445–462
16. Schapiro B (1931) Ist der Kryptorchismus chirurgisch oder hormonell zu behandeln? Dtsch Med Wochenschr 57:718
17. Rost F (1933) Versuche zum Descensus testiculorum. Langenbecks Arch Chir 177:680–684
18. Wells LJ (1943) Descent of the testis: Anatomical and hormonal considerations. Recent Adv Surg 14:436–472
19. Bergh A, Helander FH, Wahlqvist WL (1978) Studies on factors governing testicular descent in the rat, particularly the role of gubernaculum testis. Int J Androl 1:342–356
20. Wensing CJG (1973b) Testicular descent in some domestic mammals. III. Search for the factors that regulate

the gubernacular reaction. Proc Kon Ned Akad Wetensch C. 76:196–202
21. Martins T (1938) La testostérone peut provoquer la des-
   cente de testicules artificiels de paraffine. CR Soc Biol
   (Paris) 131:299–302
22. Backhouse MK (1981) Embryology of the normal and
   cryptorchid testis. In: Fonkalsrud WE, Mengel W (eds)
   Undescended testis. Year Book Med Publ, Chicago
   London
23. Elder SJ, Isaacs TJ, Walsh CP (1981) Androgenic sensitivity of the gubernaculum testis: Evidence for hormonal mechanical interactions in testicular descent. 76th
   annual meeting AUA, Boston, May 10–14, 1981.
24. Gier HT, Marion GB (1969) Development of mammalian testes and genital ducts. Biol Reprod [Suppl 1] 1–23

25. Bedford M (1978) Anatomical evidence for epididymis
   as a prime mover in the evolution of the scrotum. Am
   J Anat 152:483–507
26. Mainwaring WIP (1977) The mechanism of action of
   androgens. Springer, New York Heidelberg Berlin
27. Darwin C (1871) The descent of man and selection in
   relation to sex. J Murray, London
28. Ohno S (1979) Major sex-determining genes. Springer,
   Berlin Heidelberg New York
29. Portmann A (1965) Einführung in die vergleichende
   Morphologie der Wirbeltiere. Beno Schwabe, Basel
   Stuttgart
30. Honacki JH, Kinman KE, Koeppl JW (1982) Mammal
   species of the world. Allen Press, Kansas

3 Embryology of Testicular Descent and Maldescent

F. Hadžiselimović

During the development of the male genital tract two different stages can be discerned:

1. The initial stage is generally called an indifferent stage, lasting until the end of the 6th week after conception [1]. In this period the male and female genital tracts develop similarly, so that at the end of this phase both male and female embryos have an urogenital anlage with Wolffian and Müllerian ducts.
2. The second stage commences at the 7th week post conception (p.c.) and is clearly recognizable at the 8th week p.c. [2, 3]. This is the period when the differentiation of the testes, the epididymis, and the external genitalia occurs.

Soon after fertilization, gonadal sex is determined through the expression of H-Y antigen which induces testicular development in the gonadal anlage [4]. This was proved by the experiments of Ohno et al. [4]. When undifferentiated XX gonads of fetal calves were exposed to H-Y antigen, "complete" testicular transformation was noted. It began with the sudden appearance of the tubulus seminiferus after 3 days and culminated in the appearance of a tunica albuginea after 5 days [4]. The XX cells of the induced tubulus resemble postpubertal Sertoli cells [4]. Neither Leydig cells nor germ cells were observed [4]. The H-Y may exist in at least three different stages:

a) Bound to its specific receptor
b) As a part of the plasma membrane
c) As a free gene solution [5]

It may be inferred that the testicular organization of the indifferent gonad is secondary to the synthesis and the secretion of H-Y and to the engagement of the H-Y and its specific receptors [5]. Evidently, these events signal a programme of differentiation in Sertoli cells with a consequent formation of tubuli seminiferi, as well as to the differentiation of the Leydig cells [4]. It is evident from recent experiments that there must be a threshold of H-Y expression above which the testis is induced and below which it is not [5].

In the last few years, a three-gene hypothesis stating that a structural gene for H-Y antigen is located at an autosome has been proposed [6]. This structural gene is suspected to be under the activating or repressing influence of two genes linked with the Y and X chromosomes [6].

3.1 Indifferent Stage of Gonadal Development

The classical theory about the structural formation of the sexually indifferent gonad states that superficial epithelium through its proliferation invades the mesenchymal cord and gives rise to the primary sex cords [7]. In males these should represent the precursors of the definitive tubulus seminiferus. However, an opposing viewpoint stating that gonadal blastema is derived from mesenchymal blastema without the participation of superficial epithelium has been proposed [8]. On the other hand, Witschi postulated an inductor theory of sex differentiation [9, 10] whereby the blastemas (superficial and mesonephrogenic) influence one another, and either the cortex or medulla are given preference to building the female-cortical or male-medullary structure [9, 10]. Wartenberg further advocated that during the indifferent period mesonephrogenic cells invade the superficial epithelium [11]. The mesonephrogenic and epitheliogenic cells then intermingle [11]. They include the migrating germ cells and the final composition of the genital ridge consists of a common blastema (primary blastema) which shows no separation in two distinctive primordia [11]. The gonadal blastema gives medullary plates (precursors of the testicular cords) and serves as a reservoir for all types of testicular cells [11]. The origin of the blastema cells can be traced back to two different structures of the mesonephros:

a) Cells of a Bowman's capsule

b) Podocytes of the glomeruli [11]

The gonadal blastema is excentrically located and the "rete" blastema connects the gonadal blastema and/or the mesonephros with those parts of the testes already filled with testicular cords [11]. They deliver additional blastema cells to this area [11]. The rete blastema consists of dark mesonephrogenic cells and a lesser number of light cells [11]. In the interstitium they transform into the Leydig and peritubular cells, while in the proximal segment of the testicular cord they give rise to the Sertoli cells [11].

3.2 Differentiation of the Testis

At the 8th week p.c. the tunica albuginea, which is formed from the mesenchyme, forms septa and divides the testis into testicular lobes. In each lobe the testicular cord differentiates into two or three definitive strands, the latter of which is surrounded by a basal membrane.

3.2.1 Germ Cells

The human germ cells are first recognizable among the endodermal cells of the caudal portion of the yolk sac, near the allantoid stalk [1]. During the 5th week they migrate and reach the angle of the mesentery and the mesonephros [1]. This migration occurs in an ameboid manner [1]. The stimulus which triggers these cells to migrate is unknown. It has been shown that in amphibians the presence of either the Wolffian ducts or the notochord is necessary for genital ridge formation and the normal migration of the germ cells. Germ cells from an embryo with dorsal mesoderm and neural tube removed will migrate into the gonadal site of a normal parabiotic twin embryo [12]. In the opinion of Witschi the coelomic epithelium in the area of the gonadal anlage releases specific chemical substances which penetrate the mesenchyme, causing movement of gonocytes towards the site of greatest concentration of these hypothetical substances [10]. Falin's study [1] corroborates the theory of the extragonadal origin of primordial germ cells and of their direct participation in the formation of definitive germ cells. The process of differentiation of the gonocytes (primordial germ cells) and their transformation begins later in males than in females. The cytoplasm of these primordial germ cells contains a large amount of glycogen and there is a definite interdependence between the accumulation of glycogen in the germ cells and the process of differentiation [1, 14].

The primordial cells are observable up to 145 days p.c. [14]. In the testes they transform into gonocytes [13]. Fukuda et al. further differentiate an additional type called the intermedial type of germ cell, which develops from gonocytes and gives rise to the fetal spermatogonium [13]. Until the 10th week p.c., most of the germ cells belong to the gonocyte type. Around the 15th week, the intermedial cell becomes predominant while the gonocytes are still present [13]. After the 22nd week p.c. most of the germ cells should be fetal spermatogonia and the typical gonocytes are almost absent [13]. Observations on our collection of the fetal testes from the 28th week of pregnancy confirmed the presence of fetal spermatogonia and two types of gonocytes. The ultrastructural appearance of the gonocytes can be described as follows: The major part of the cells is occupied by a round nucleus which has one or two centrally located nucleoli. The chromatin forms small clumps and is less dispersed than that of a fetal spermatogonia. Occasionally, a protrusion can be observed on the nuclear membrane. This cup-like formation is a marked lifting of the nuclear membrane from the structure with a cavity in the interior and is evidently a normal phenomenon. Such nuclear protuberances can also be observed in gonocytes where no signs of any degeneration are visible. This structure on the nucleus is connected with the appearance of so-called chromatid bodies, which are frequently present in the cytoplasm of fetal spermatogonia. The narrow cytoplasm contains a relatively large number of the small round mitochondria of the tubulus type (Fig. 1a). These are larger than those of the Sertoli cells, and as a rule do not form any intermitochondrial substance. A large number of polyribosomes and glycogen granules are visible in the cytoplasm. Their rough endoplasmic reticulum and the smooth endoplasmic reticulum are very sparse. The pseudopodia-like processus, which extends towards the periphery, contains micropinocytotic vesicles. A second type of gonocyte,

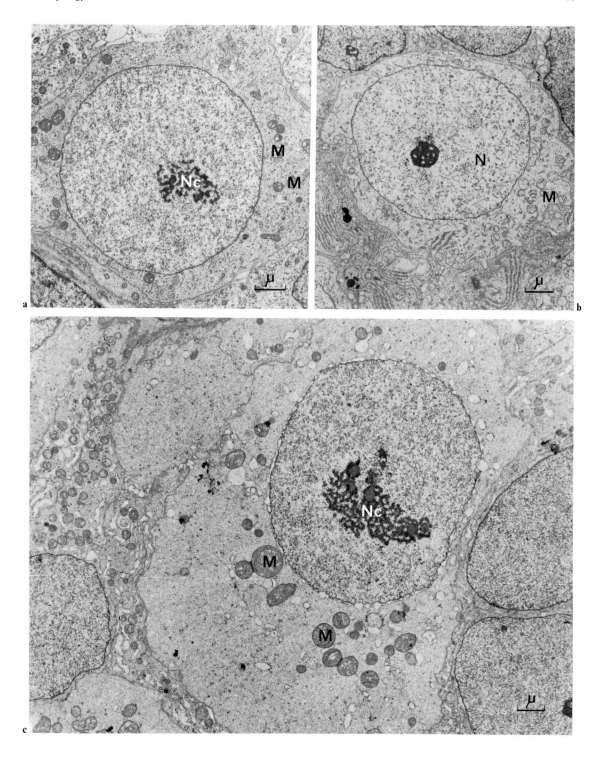

Fig. 1. a Gonocyte type 1, with large centrally located nucleolus (*Nc*). The mitochondria (*M*) are generally smaller than those of fetal spermatogonia and of the tubule type. **b** Gonocyte type 2, with a pale cytoplasm and a pale nucleus (*N*). **c** The fetal spermatogonium, besides having the larger cell size, has a pale cytoplasm and a large mitochondria of the tubule type (*M*). The nucleolus (*Nc*) is reticular and centrally located

generally smaller and with the nucleolus and cytoplasm displaced in favour of the nucleus, also exists in the fetal tubulus seminiferus (Fig. 1 b). The cytoplasm is electron-light with a small amount of rough endoplasmic reticulum and a crista-type mitochondria. Glycogen is completely lacking in the cytoplasm of this gonocyte. The protrusion of pseudopodia, which, in the first type of gonocytes described above, are directed towards the basement membrane, are here only rudimentary, or completely absent. From the ultrastructural point of view, these cells may be said to correspond to the so-called intermediate cells [13]. The assumption that the latter cells are gonocytes which will be phagocytized by Sertoli cells is supported by the fact that they cells are found mainly in the center of the tubulus and possess no or only very rudimentary pseudopodia and a narrow, light cytoplasm with signs of degenerating mitochondria [15] (Fig. 1 b).

The histological appearance and general characteristics of the fetal spermatogonia are widely accepted [13, 15, 16]. This cell is the largest cell within the fetal and child's tubulus seminiferus. It is always in contact with the basement membrane [16, 17]. The cytoplasm is noticeably transparent. The form of the nucleus is round to oval and it is about twice as large as that of the neighboring Sertoli cell. In the middle of the nucleus lies a large nucleolus, consisting of a loose reticular substance and two to three amorphous bodies (Fig. 1c). The chromatin is homogeneously dispersed over the entire nucleus. A typical feature of the fetal spermatogonia is a large mitochondria (Fig. 1c). They are connected with the intermitochondrial substance. The mitochondria are mainly of the tubular type, but also some of a crista type can be found. The Golgi complex and the rough as well as the smooth endoplasmic reticulum are sparsely distributed. The chromatid bodies are frequently observed in the vicinity of the nucleus. In 1974 an attempt was made to unify the terminology of germ cell development, but this was based on the studies

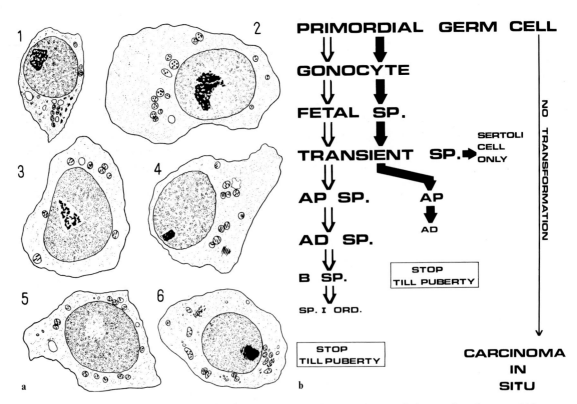

Fig. 2. a Different types of children's germ cells: *1* gonocyte; *2* fetal spermatogonium; *3* transient spermatogonium; *4* AP spermatogonium; *5* AD spermatogonium; *6* B spermatogonium. **b** The development and transformation of the germ cells in normal testes (*light arrow*) and cryptorchid testes (*dark arrow*). The hypothetical nontransformation of primordial germ cells may lead to the development of carcinoma in situ

on rats [18]. The following description of germ cell development was suggested: Primordial germ cells give rise to M prospermatogonia, which transform into T2 prospermatogonia via the T1 prospermatogonia stage. From T2 prospermatogonia the adult spermatogonia differentiate [18]. The major problem of this classification is that it does not include all the cell types observed in the human testis throughout embryonal life and childhood, as described above and in Chap. 4.

According to our results and recent relevant publications it can be concluded that: Primordial cells differentiate in the gonocytes by entering the testicular cords. The gonocytes attached to the basement membrane give rise to the fetal spermatogonia, while the gonocytes resting in the center of the tubulus seminiferus degenerate. Fetal spermatogonia thus transform via the transitional type of spermatogonia into A-type spermatogonia. This transformation takes place after birth (Fig. 2).

3.2.2 Sertoli Cells

In the testicular cords, at the 7th week p.c., the mesenchymatous cells from the common blastema develop into the Sertoli cells [11]. They enlarge and progressively envelop the gonocytes, entering into very close contact with them. These fetal Sertoli cells have a typical appearance; they are polarized, the cell body being divided by the nucleus into basal and apical parts [13, 17]. The basal part of each cell lies along the basement membrane and is broader and shorter than the apical part. The nucleus is elliptical and has several invaginations. There is no cytoplasm "halo" surrounding the nucleus. The loose reticular nucleolus lies generally in a central position. The mitochondria, which are oval or longish in shape, are of the crista type and are found in groups in both the basal and apical parts of the cell. The Golgi apparatus is well developed, showing both lamellar and vesicular structures, and is generally situated in the vicinity of the nucleus and the apical part of the cell. A typical feature of the fetal Sertoli cells is the parallel and sometimes concentrically arranged rough endoplasmic reticulum which lies in three to six rows in the cytoplasm. It forms contacts with the lipoid droplets which occur in the basal as well as in the apical part of the cell. In addition to the rough endoplasmic reticulum, a smooth endoplasmic reticulum is also found in the cytoplasm of the Sertoli cell. The lipoid droplets can be observed particularly frequently grouped around the lamellar body [17]. This body, formed by the junction of H-shaped lamellae, is found only in the fetal and adult Sertoli cells and continues into the rough endoplasmic reticulum. Polyribosomes and glycogen are scattered throughout the cytoplasm. Between the individual Sertoli cells a complex as well as a simple "tight" cell junction can be observed. In the apical part of the cells, round bodies, which are strongly osmophilic and form clumps, can occasionally be found. Two unmistakable parts can be distinguished; a round part, centrally situated, strongly osmophilic, a relict of the nucleus of a phagocytized cell, and a granular, less osmophilic part, lying round the nucleus. The whole body is bound by a partially interrupted membrane (Fig. 3a). The consequence of digestion of these cells is a clear vacuole within the Sertoli cell cytoplasm [17].

3.2.3 Leydig Cells

From the 8th week onward the Leydig cells may be recognised within the interstitium by their characteristic shape. Electron microscopy shows a rapid augmentation of their smooth endoplasmic reticulum and mitochondria, whereas the proportion of free ribosomes and rough endoplasmic reticulum diminishes. Four different periods in the development of the Leydig cells during the fetal life can be perceived [19]:

1. The indifferent stage up to the 8th week.
2. The invading period from the 8th to the 14th week. In this period the Leydig cells encroach into the space between the testicular cords.
3. From the 14th to the 18th week the maturation phase of the interstitial cell is observed. The most predominant feature in this period is the abundance of smooth endoplasmic reticulum in the cytoplasm of the fetal Leydig cells [19].
4. From the 18th week until the 2nd year of life degeneration and diminution of the Leydig cells occur [17, 19].

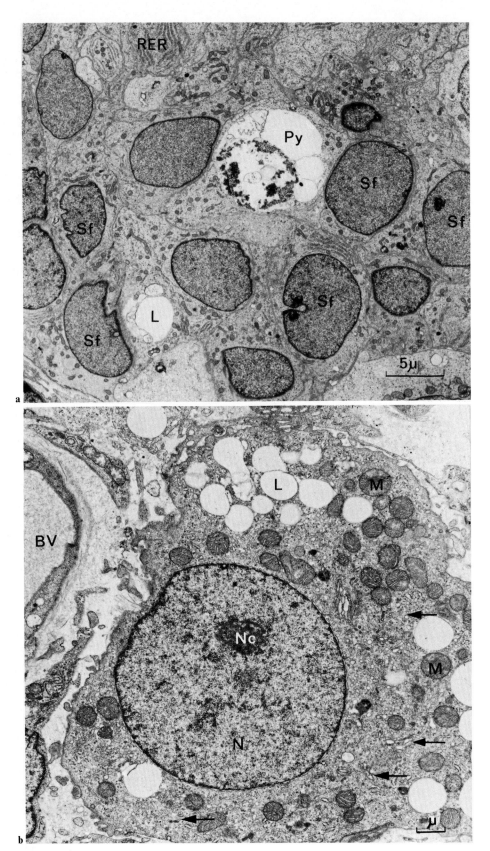

From the 28th week p.c. the Leydig cells are frequently observed lying together in small groups within the interstitium. Between the cells there is an intercellular cleft about 150 Å in diameter. A direct contact between the Leydig cells and blood vessels is not observed either in fetal or in children's interstitium. At their surface, the Leydig cells are only partially covered by the basement membrane. Fetal Leydig cells measure about 30 µm. A prominent feature is their round nucleus with two or three nucleoli lying eccentrically. The heterochromatin is predominantly connected with the nuclear membrane. The cytoplasm is mainly composed of mitochondria, Golgi apparatus, cytosomes, ribosomes, and smooth endoplasmic reticulum. The form of the mitochondria varies considerably and there are tubular as well as a crista type of mitochondria observable. The Golgi apparatus is usually situated in the vicinity of the nucleus. The rare ribosomes are organized as polysomes but occasionally they develop contact with the smooth endoplasmic reticulum. The lipoid droplets are scattered all around the cytoplasm and there is a close contact between them, the smooth endoplasmic reticulum, and the mitochondria (Fig. 3 b).

3.3 Male Duct Differentiation and Development

During the 4th week p.c. the mesonephros is derived from the intermediate mesoderm and is located on the posterior abdominal wall within a longitudinal mass of mesenchyme, which projects downwards into the coelomic cavity. In the male, the greatest extent of the mesonephros is from the second thoracic vertebral segment to the second lumbar vertebral segment [20]. The fold of parietal peritoneum over the mesonephros has a maximal extent from the fourth cervical vertebral segment to the fourth lumbar vertebral segment [20]. This me-

sonephric fold covers the ventral aspect of the mesonephros [20]. With the organization of the testes the differentiation and formation of the excretory duct take place. This is accomplished by the transformation of the Wolffian duct and the mesonephric tubulus into the epididymis, ductus deferens, and seminal vesicle. The organization of the Wolffian duct is dependent on androgen produced by the Leydig cells, and the regression of the Müllerian duct is dependent on the factor or hormone presumably produced by the fetal Sertoli cells and called Müllerian inhibiting substance (MIS) [21]. The entire duct system in the mammal consists of tubulus seminiferus, rete tubule, vasa efferentia, epididymis, vas deferens, and urethra.

In a 43 mm C.R. human male embryo (10.5 weeks), the mesonephros, which is holding the testis like a forceps, bears in its upper section part of a mesonephric tubule (Fig. 4). The formation of this tubule begins at the cephalic pole of the mesonephros. The processus vaginalis is recognizable as a small invagination at the level of the deep inguinal ring (Figs. 4, 5). The inguinal canal, which was thus formed at 16 mm C.R. [22], is filled with gubernacular mesenchyma (Fig. 5). Two ligaments can be encountered as a continuation of the mesonephros; cranially the diaphragmatic ligament and caudally the gubernaculum. The plica vascularis should be considered as distinct from the diaphragmatic ligament. Cranially the gubernaculum insertion is the Wolffian duct and caudally it extends into the inguinal canal. This gubernaculum mass remains within the inguinal canal (Fig. 5). There is no direct contact between the testis and the gubernaculum. The testis has at this stage of development completed the change in its shape from elliptical into rounder formation (Figs. 4, 5).

At 90 mm C.R. (around 14 weeks p.c.) important changes have occurred within the mesonephros. Its upper part is still in continuation with the dorsal abdominal wall over a thread-like elongated diaphragmatic ligament. The cranial portion of the epididymis starts to develop. Here the coiling of the Wolffian duct is clearly recognizable at this stage of development. In the caudal part of the mesonephros, a condensation of mesenchymal tissue takes place and this occurs mainly within the gubernaculum. The processus vaginalis is deeper and broader while the testis has a round shape (Fig. 4).

Fig. 3. a The fetal Sertoli cells (*Sf*), abundant rough endoplasmic reticulum (*RER*), large vacuole (*L*), and phagocytotic vacuole (*Py*). **b** The fetal Leydig cell with a smooth endoplasmic reticulum (*arrows*), lipoid droplets (*L*) and various-shaped mitochondria (*M*). Leydig cell is placed in the vicinity of the blood vessel (*Bv*)

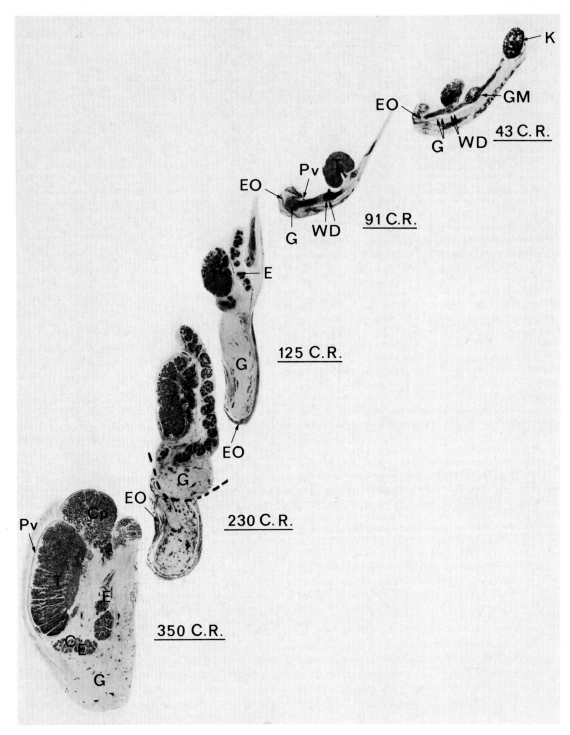

Fig. 4. Photomontage of testicular descent in man from 43 mm to 350 mm C.R. presented in a sagittal plane. The gubernaculum (*G*) at 43 mm and 90 mm is mesenchymatous and never penetrating through the external abdominal muscle fascia (*EO*). Proximally it inserts into the Wolffian duct (*WD, double arrow*) or in the epididymis (*E*). From the 125 mm stage it enlarges and develops its ground substance similar to that of Wharton's jelly of the umbilicus. The continuous development of the epididymis, particularly the increase in its tortuosity parallel to the degree of testicular displacement, is evident. At 230 mm the caput epididymidis (*Cp*) enfolds the testis and remains thus for the remainder of descent. The *interrupted line* divides the gubernaculum into two parts. In reality, the lower one is situated more medially. Kidney (*K*), glomerule of mesonephros (*GM*), cauda epididymidis (*C_E*), Testis (*T*)

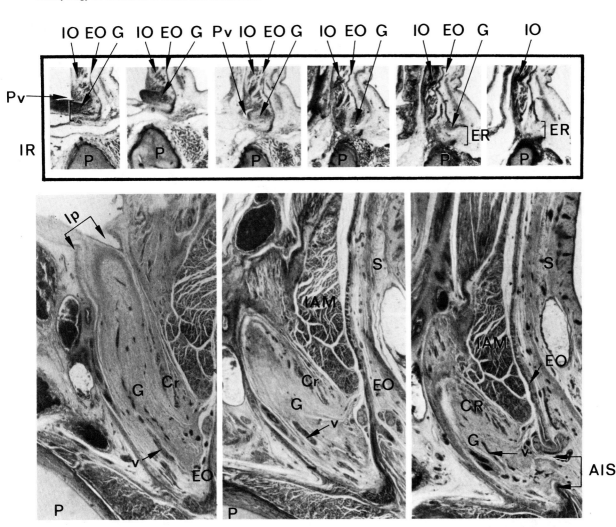

Fig. 5. a The gubernaculum (*G*) and the processus vaginalis of a 45 mm C.R. human embryo, (*Pv*) are thus to be followed from the deep inguinal ring (*IR*) to the superficial inguinal ring (*ER*). The gubernaculum terminates at the superficial inguinal ring without continuing into the scrotum. The development of the testis coverings is still in progress. The fascia of the external abdominal oblique muscle (*EO*), the internal abdominal oblique muscle (*IO*), and the pubis (*P*) are shown. **b** Three different sagittal sections of a 125 mm C.R. human embryo. A proximal section through the internal inguinal pouch (*Ip*) shows the jelly-like ground substance of the gubernaculum (*G*). Within the gubernaculum an increased vascularization (*V*) is observable. At the periphery of the gubernaculum, the cremaster fibers (*Cr*) are evidently derived from the internal abdominal oblique muscle (*IAM*). At the level of the superficial inguinal pouch (*AIS*) no direct continuation of the gubernaculum into the scrotum is discernible. External oblique fascia (*EO*), pubis (*P*), skin (*S*)

Three weeks later, at 125 mm C.R., the position of the gonad is at the deep inguinal ring. The transabdominal movement of the testis is terminated. This motion is not as distinct as in rodents because of pelvis configuration, but becomes distinguishable if the comparison between 90 mm C.R. and 125 mm C.R. in sagittal plane is made (Fig. 4). With the disappearance of the diaphragmatic ligament, the erection of the long testis diameter into the vertical axis has occurred. Three portions of the epididymis are recognisable, namely, the caput, the cauda and the corpus epididymidis. The epididymis now completely surrounds the testis (Fig. 4). The gubernaculum is relatively longer and broader, its diameter equalling that of the gonad. Its transparent structure is recognizable within the inguinal canal. The ground sub-

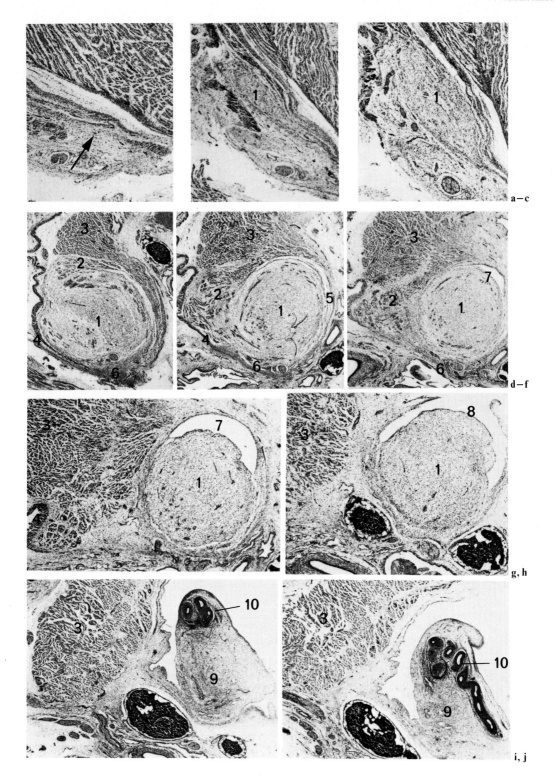

stance of the gubernaculum resembles that of the Wharton's jelly in the umbilical cord (Figs. 5, 6). At the periphery of the inguinal part of the gubernaculum, the musculus cremaster fibers are observable. The musculus cremaster is adjacent to the internal abdominal muscle, giving an impression of being derived from it (Figs. 5, 6). No encroachment into the central gubernacular substance by the musculus cremaster is observable (Figs. 4, 5, 6). No balloon-like swelling of the gubernaculum occurs, and nor did any distinct expansion of the gubernaculum outside the inguinal canal take place (Figs. 5, 6).

The relationship between the diameter of the gubernaculum and the diameter of the testis remains constant up to 230 mm C.R. (around 26 weeks p.c.) (Fig. 4). The position of the gonad is still at the annulus inguinalis profundus. The absolute dimensions of both testes and gubernaculum have increased. At this stage, around the distal part of the gubernaculum, some muscle fibers are encountered. These fibers have a circular arrangement (Figs. 4, 6). The epididymis is further developed and the caput epididymidis now lies adjacent to the testis (Fig. 4). Compared to 125 mm C.R., the gubernacular ground substance at this stage is better interwoven by blood vessels (Figs. 4, 6c).

The gubernaculum does not herniate the abdominal wall. As has recently been stated, the abdominal wall structure develops round it in the inguinal canal and later in the scrotum [22].

At 350 mm C.R. (40 weeks p.c.) testicular descent is terminated. The testis now lies within

---

Fig. 6a–j. Frontal serial sections of the inguinal canal of a 16-week-old male fetus. **a** The superficial inguinal pouch is narrow (*arrow*) and there is no gubernacular continuation into the scrotum. × 10. **b** In the next deeper layers the mesenchymatous mass of the gubernaculum (*1*) appears. × 10. **c** The gubernacular mass, lacking cremaster fibers, is progressively enlarging. Its shape is still elliptical. × 10. **d** At the periphery of the now round gubernaculum cross section the cremaster fibers (*2*), being a continuation of the internal abdominal muscle (*3*), are recognizable. × 10. **e** Topography of the inguinal canal: in front, the aponeurosis of the external oblique fascia (*4*); behind, the transversalis fascia (*5*); above, the arched fibers of the internal oblique and transverse abdominal muscles (*3*); below, the inguinal ligament (*6*). × 10. **f** The processus vaginalis (*7*) appears. × 10. **g** Frontal section close to the deep inguinal pouch. × 15. **h** Internal inguinal ponch (*8*) × 15. **i, j** The intra-abdominal part of the gubernaculum (*9*) inserting into the cauda epididymidis (*10*) × 15

---

the scrotum (Fig. 4). An increase in the vascularization of the gubernaculum is recognizable and it shrinks. A considerable amount of collagen is now scattered throughout the mesenchyma ground substance of the gubernaculum (Fig. 7a). The cauda epididymidis has attained its final shape and lies in close contact with the inferior pole of the testis (Fig. 4). The L formation of the epididymis, as already visible at 220 mm C.R., is still present (Figs. 4, 8). The caput epididymidis has also reached its final shape, lying close to the upper testicular pole. Both ductuli efferentes, as well as the Wolffian duct, take part in the formation of the caput epididymidis.

The continuous development of the epididymis throughout the whole descent contrasts with the published observation that the cauda epididymidis invades the gubernacular mesenchyma at the end of testicular descent [22].

3.3.1 Development of the Testis Coverings

The testis is situated intraperitoneally throughout the whole descent. This position is clearly recognisable at 43 mm C.R., 91 mm C.R., and 125 mm C.R. At the end of testicular descent the caput and a part of the cauda lie intraperitoneally, while the gubernaculum, the cauda epididymidis, and the greater part of the corpus are retroperitoneal. As the abdominal muscle begins to differentiate around the 16 mm C.R., [22] the transverse fascia gives rise to the tunica spermatica interna, while the cremaster muscle was described as being in loop separated from the lower margin of the internal oblique muscle. This generally accepted development of the cremaster muscle is categorically rejected by Backhouse [22]. He observed a completely new muscle differentiation into the cremaster muscle from the inguinal ligament (lateral cremaster) and the pubis (medial cremaster), extending into the periphery of the gubernacular mesenchyma within the inguinal region. The different innervation (genitofemoral nerve) than the obliquus internus (ilioinguinal nerve) and the different local myopathic lesions were additional evidence stated by Backhouse for the identity of the cremaster muscle [22]. The innervation of the cremaster muscle is however not generally accepted as being from the genitofemoral nerve; the ilioinguinal nerve is also thought to

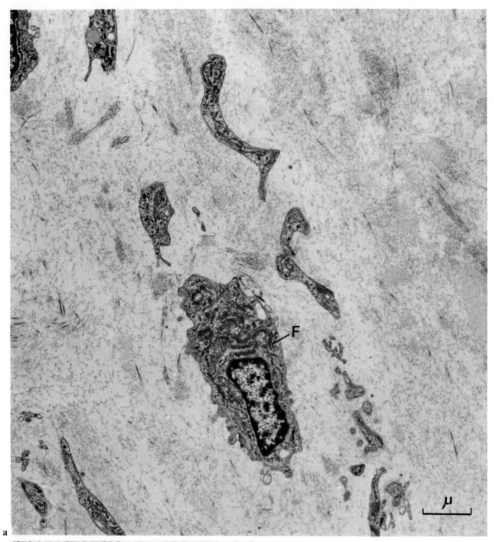

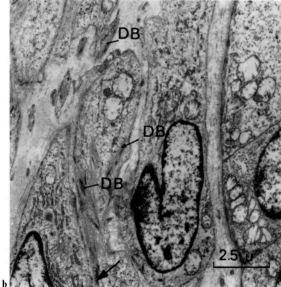

Fig. 7. a An electron-microscopic view of the gubernaculum in the newborn. Fibroblasts (*F*) are loosely distributed within the ground substance. No muscle fibers are perceptible. **b** The myofibroblasts around the ductus of the epididymis of a 26-week-old human male fetus. The typical features of the myofibroblast are a dense body (*DB*) and a gap junction (*arrow*)

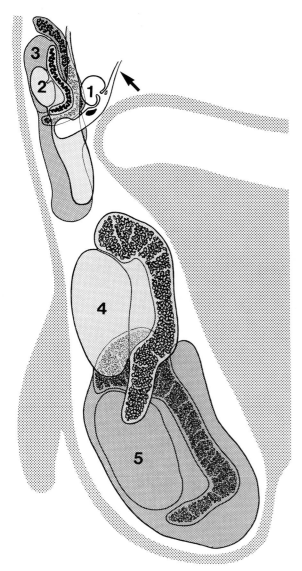

Fig. 8. Testicular descent in man: 90 mm$_{CR}$ (*1*); 125 mm$_{CR}$ (*2*); 230 mm$_{CR}$ (*3*); 280 mm$_{CR}$ (*4*); at term (*5*). The transabdominal movement is clearly perceived between 90 mm and 125 mm$_{CR}$. In this period the diaphragmatic ligament (*arrow*) disappears and the testis is erected to an upright position. The differentiation of the epididymis parallels the degree of testicular descent. The epididymis always precedes the testis. × 5

ternal oblique muscle. This fascia, particularly in older fetuses when the separation zone is pronounced, completely surrounds the gubernaculum, so that there is no direct contact between the gubernaculum and the scrotal wall.

3.3.2 Comparison of Testicular Descent in Humans and Rodents

As testicular descent is an event occurring in both rodents and humans, their similarities should help us to understand this mechanism. The timing of testicular descent and the need for an inguinal canal are not prerequisites; both differ between the human and the mouse. Further, the structure of the gubernaculum is different; fibrous in rodents, jelly mesenchymatous in man. Rodents have a conus inguinalis, yet no such structure is found during the ontogenetic development within the gubernaculum in man. Neither in mouse nor in man has any swelling of the gubernaculum been observed throughout the whole descent. While in man the testis and the epididymis sink into the ground substance of the gubernaculum, this does not happen in the mouse (Figs. 4, 8, 9). The craniocaudal direction of the epididymis differentiation and the coiling of the epididymis is identical for both species. Both species have the same cranial insertion of the gubernaculum, namely the Wolffian duct and later in the developing cauda epididymidis. In both species testicular descent occurs intra-abdominally within the processus vaginalis peritonei. The changes in the testis shape are similar in both species, indicating that these changes may have some additional influence on the process of testicular descent. The importance of the epididymis in testicular descent becomes apparent if we realize the mode of differentiation (in both species), the enlargement of the cauda in the crucial phase of descent, and in general, the coiling of the epididymis. In both species, changes in the center of gravitation due to the craniocaudal differentiation of the epididymis influence testicular descent significantly. The secretion of the fluid, within a differentiating Wolffian duct, develops a stronger pressure at the center of gravity and helps to change the position of the epididymis and passively the position of the testis, as the latter is carried by the epididymis. The ultrastructural examinations of human em-

be a motor nerve to the muscle [23]. The intimate proximity of the cremaster muscle with the internal abdominal oblique muscle throughout the whole development indicates that the latter muscle may be the origin of the former (Figs. 4, 5, 6). The tunica spermatica externa is generally accepted to be derived from the ex-

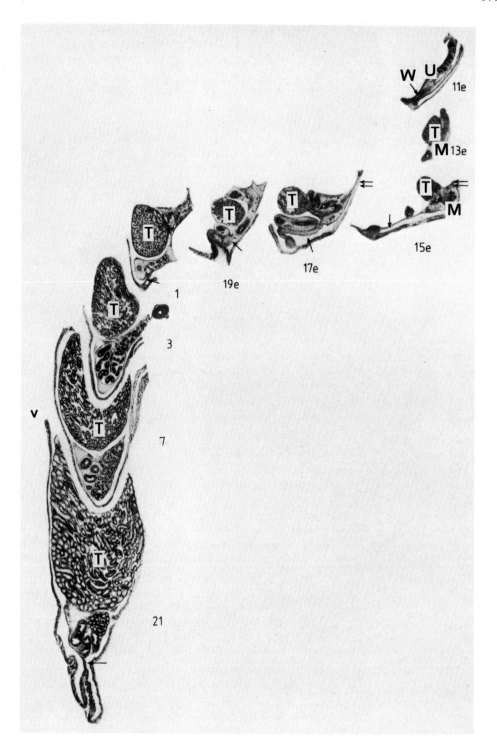

Fig. 9. Photomontage of testicular descent in the mouse. The course of descent is S-shaped from dorsal-superior to ventral-inferior. 11th, 13th, 15th, 17th, and 19th days of gestation and 1st, 3rd, 7th, and 21st days after birth are shown. The urogenital anlage (*U*), Wolffian duct (*W*), testis (*T*), mesonephros (*M*) and gubernaculum (*arrow*) can be followed in their ontogenetic development. The magnifica-tion of all stages is the same (× 13.5) so the relative development of gonadal growth and craniocaudal epididymis and ductus deferens differentiation is comparable. Note: the gubernaculum never inserts directly into the testis, and there is no extra-abdominal swelling of the gubernaculum. Marked testicular enlargement starts postnatally. *Double arrow* = diafragmatic ligament

bryonal mesenchymal cells which are concentrically arranged around the Wolffian duct show the existence of filaments of ca. 60 Å thickness in their cytoplasm, a typical feature of the myofibroblasts (Fig. 7b). It is well known that in rats the first peristaltic motion of the Wolffian duct is already observed in early embryonal life [24]. This early movement of the Wolffian duct, together with the fluid pressure which develops in the craniocaudally differentiating epididymis, may have an important influence on testicular descent. The processus vaginalis, although not the main factor, is surely a prerequisite for normal testicular descent. It enables the testis to reach the scrotum through the inguinal canal with a minimum of friction. Testicular descent itself is independent of the descent of the processus vaginalis. The testis neither pushes the processus vaginalis down in its descent, nor is pulled down by it.

3.4 Estrogen-Induced Cryptorchidism

In a strain of mutant mice with hypogonadism due to a GnRH deficiency, the involvement of the hypothalamo-pituitary-gonadal axis in the pathogenesis of cryptorchidism was obvious [25]. Apart from being cryptorchid these mice were sterile [25].

The application of estradiol to pregnant rodents represents the most singular experiment in the research of cryptorchidism, even to this day. Using estradiol it was possible to induce the development of a cryptorchid state without having to resort to surgery [26].

Further experiments with antiandrogens (cyproterone acetate and its derivatives) produced differing results (27, 28). While some researchers found that cyproterone acetate inhibited testicular descent [27], others observed no effect [28]. Wensing and co-workers [29], who initially believed that the "swelling reaction" of the gubernaculum was androgen-dependent, later revised their opinion after experimentation with cyproterone acetate [30]. An attempt to induce the swelling reaction of the gubernaculum with androgens in female pigs has also failed. In contrast, a partial descent of the ovaries has been observed in freemartins. In immature monkeys [31] and opossums [32] it was possible to achieve premature descent with the application of androgens.

Since Raynaud [33] not only inhibited descent with estrogen, but also induced partial persistence of the Müllerian duct, the hypothesis arose in later years, that it is not androgen but the Müllerian inhibiting substance (MIS) which may be responsible for descent [34]. However, the fact that in the majority of cryptorchid animals and humans no remnants of the Müllerian duct were observable unmistakably contradicts the hypothesis that MIS is the main factor in testicular descent. Also, the factors against MIS involvement in achieving testicular descent stem from the observation that testicular descent could be terminated after the 2nd year of life, the period when MIS is no longer produced [35].

To prove the role of the hypothalamo-pituitary-gonadal axis in the pathogenesis of cryptorchidism, Swiss albino mice were treated with estradiol or estradiol and HCG [36, 38]. Cryptorchidism was achieved in 75%–100% of all estradiol-treated male mice. Not only bilateral, but also unilateral cryptorchidism was found. The Leydig cells of estradiol-treated mice displayed atrophic characteristics which were previously observed in cryptorchid newborns [37]. The testosterone content of cryptorchid mice testes was 49 pg/testis, whereas the newborn controls had a testosterone content of 106 pg/testis ($P < 0.001$). The weight of newborn E_2B mice testes (1.29 mg) and that of the control mice (1.23 mg) was not significantly different. In adult mice treated with estradiol during intrauterine life, the ultrastructural changes in the Leydig cells also show severe signs of atrophy [38]. The testosterone content of the testes of these adult mice was 0.07 ng/mg, compared to 0.53 ng/mg in controls ($P < 0.001$).

The higher the position of the gonad, the more marked the changes in the mesonephros [39]. In cryptorchid mice, the testes remained in the dorsal position and there was no intra-abdominal migration. In cases where it did happen, this process was not complete [40]. The transformation of the Wolffian duct into the ductus deferens and the epididymis was also incomplete and the tubules of the Wolffian duct appeared much more enlarged and reduced in number [39, 40]. In the mesenchyma itself, considerable changes occurred. There was a substantial increase in the number of mesenchymal cells positioned concentrically around the individual tubule of the Wolffian duct. The entire

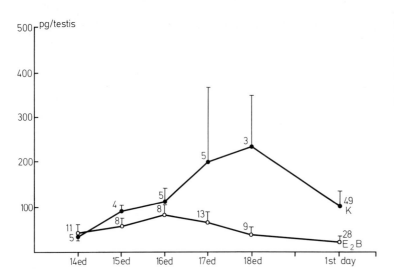

Fig. 10. Testicular testosterone through-out the embryonal life of the mouse. Control (*K*) mice display a sharp increase in testicular testosterone around the 17th and 18th embryonal days (*Ed*). This is completely lacking in estrogen-treated cryptorchid mice (E₂B)

mesonephros appeared broader, while the gubernaculum was narrower [39, 40].

Administration of estrogen hindered the transformation of the Wolffian duct. This should not be regarded as resulting from a direct effect of estrogen on the mesonephros, but rather as a consequence of androgen deficiency brought about by an insufficient stimulation of the Leydig cells by gonadotropin (Fig. 10). The testicles of mice treated simultaneously with HCG and E_2B were capable of completing descensus. The lower the position of the testicles the better differentiated were the ductus deferens and the epididymis [40].

Based on the position of the testes in E_2B and HCG-treated mice, two distinct groups can be identified, namely descended and undescended. The descended group had a mean testicular testosterone of 129 pg/testis compared to 90 pg/testis in the cryptorchid group (2 $\alpha = 0.01$ Wilcoxon test). This indicated that the testicular testosterone level had to be sufficiently high to induce the transformation of the Wolffian duct into the epididymis and thus descent (Fig. 11 a–c). The recent findings on estradiol-treated immature rats confirmed our observations [41]. It was also possible to prevent cryptorchidism by the simultaneous administration of HCG and dihydrotestosterone, indicating that dihydrotestosterone may be the hormone essential for testicular descent [41].

3.5 Spontaneous Congenital Cryptorchidism in Mice: Treatment with GnRH

Six to nine percent of Charles River strain of mice had congenitally uni- or bilateral cryptorchidism. These mice were sterile [40]. The testicular testosterone level was significantly lower when compared to the controls (Fig. 12). The Leydig cells of these mice were atrophic. GnRH treatment of 14 days duration with 5 µg daily i.m. led to bilateral descent in 60% of the mice. In 13% (2/15) there was unilateral descent and in 27% (4/15) descent did not occur. After GnRH treatment the testosterone level in the cryptorchid testes rose significantly (Fig. 12) [40, 42]. Testicular weight remained the same, indicating that it did not have an important role in inducing testicular descent (Fig. 12). The main changes occurred in the length of the epididymis of the cryptorchid group. Before treat-

Fig. 11 a–c. The 17th embryonal day. **a** in control male mice; **b** in estrogen-treated mice; **c** in mice treated with a combination of estrogen and HCG. While in the estrogen-treated mice the testes (*I*) remained in the neighborhood of the kidney (*K*), the testes in the other two groups are already in the vicinity of the ventral abdominal wall (*V*). The essential difference between the cryptorchid group and the other two groups is that the former displays a rudimentarily developed cranial part of the Wolffian duct (*WD*) (only few tubules), (*DE*). (*D*), dorsal abdominal wall, (*B*) bladder

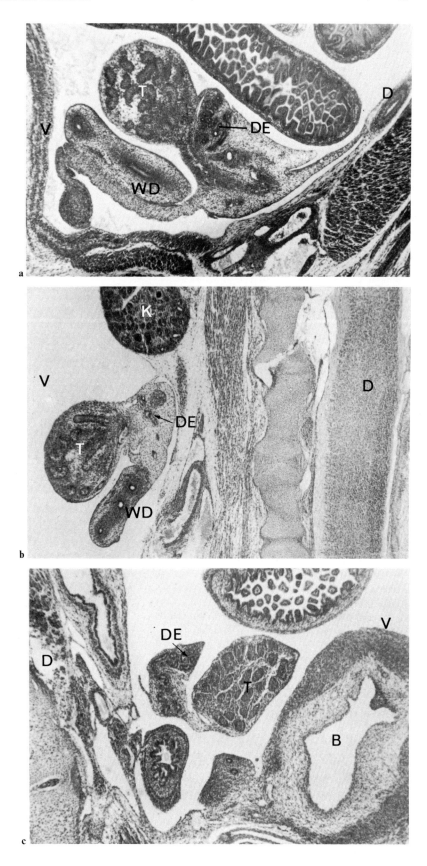

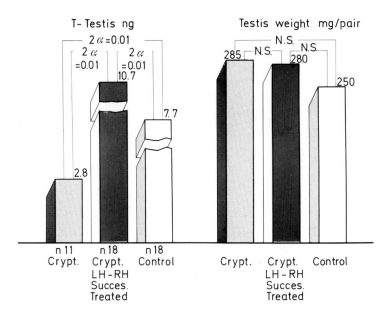

Fig. 12. Testicular weight and testosterone content in cryptorchid, successfully treated cryptorchid, and control adult male mice

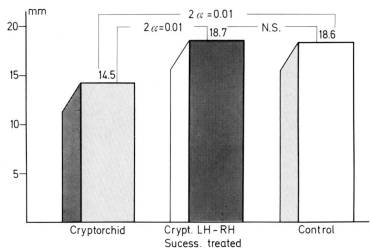

Fig. 13. The length of the epididymis in cryptorchid mice compared to the controls and successfully treated cryptorchid mice

ment it was significantly shorter, but after treatment it improved and reached the same length as the epididymis of the control animals (Fig. 13). Histologically, the cryptorchid epididymis had fewer tubules, indicating that the whole length of the ductus epididymidis is shorter. After successful treatment, the histology of the epididymis resembled that of the normal, except that the ductus epididymidis was still lacking sperm (Fig. 14). This indicates that 14 days treatment with GnRH, although inducing descent, did not significantly improve sperm production.

3.6 Morphology and Histology of the Cryptorchid Epididymis

Abnormalities in the construction of the epididymis have been encountered and described in connection with undescended testis. The most common abnormality is the looped or elongated cauda epididymidis. The other forms of abnormalities can be summarized as follows:

1. Agenesis of the testis [43]
2. Absent internal spermatic artery [44]

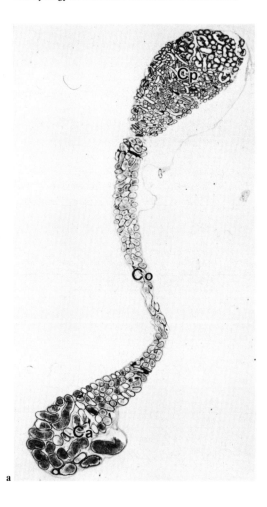
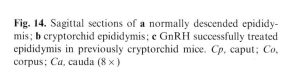
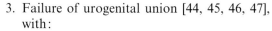
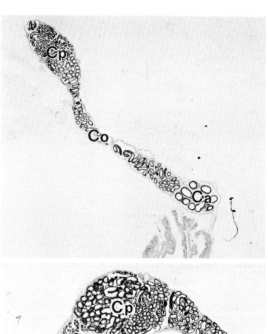
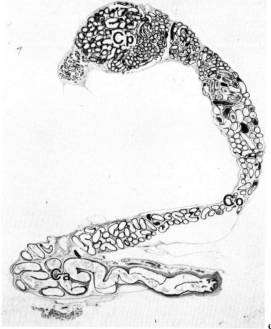

Fig. 14. Sagittal sections of **a** normally descended epididymis; **b** cryptorchid epididymis; **c** GnRH successfully treated epididymis in previously cryptorchid mice. *Cp*, caput; *Co*, corpus; *Ca*, cauda (8 ×)

3. Failure of urogenital union [44, 45, 46, 47], with:
   a) Descent of the epididymis and vas deferens
   b) Descent of the vas deferens only
   c) Partial descent of the epididymis and vas
4. Absent epididymis and vas [44, 45, 46, 47, 48]
5. Different forms of atresia:
   a) Proximal [44]
   b) Mid-epididymal [49]
   c) Distal due to atresia of Wolffian duct early in embryonal life [44]

6. Total infarction with resolution of the testis and epididymis [44]

It was estimated that unilateral testicular agenesis occurs in one of 5,000 cases and bilaterally in one of 20,000 cases [43]. However, in the case of unilateral "agenesis" where the surgeon found only an intrascrotal epididymis, the atrophic testis could be detected when serial histologic sections were performed (Fig. 15). This indicates that true agenesis may be found even more rarely than suspected.

It is important to identify the testicular vessels in all cases of inguinally or scrotally

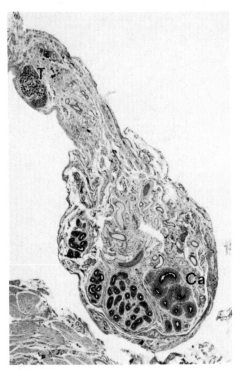

Fig. 15. The descended cauda epididymis (*Ca*) and atrophic testis (*T*) macroscopically believed to resemble anorchia (8.5×)

located vas and epididymis. If the vessels are found to accompany the vas and terminate with it, a separate testis can safely be excluded [43].

As early as 1890, Bramann stated that when there is no epididymis testicular descent cannot take place [50, 51]. In his opinion, this was due to the inability of the gubernaculum to exert traction on the testis while being directly inserted into the epididymis. Urogenital malunion early in embryonal life results in a malformed epididymal head. The testis is retained [52]. Several other investigators also pointed out that complete failure of the fusion this the testis or absence of the epididymis is always associated with cryptorchidism [45, 46].

However, there are also some reports of testicular descent lacking the epididymis [48, 53, 54]. None of these was histologically proven on the basis of serial sections, so it is not possible to distinguish if this was secondary atresia and resolution of the epididymis or a real congenital absence of the epididymis.

In a progressive study of 42 cryptorchid patients different abnormalities of the epididymis

were encountered in 36% of the cases [49]. Recently, Scorer and Farrington suggested that only 25% of undescended testes which were found in the superficial inguinal pouch and which were obstructed in their descent had a normal epididymis. The rest all tended to show some degree of epididymal abnormality [55].

All of seven cryptorchid newborns whom we examined had abnormalities of the epididymis. This was expressed in connection with the coiling of the epididymis and the development of the whole ductal system. An important observation was that the head of the epididymis, in all cases examined, was not lying on the apex of the testis. This may suggest that the positioning of the head is important to testicular descent. When the unilateral cryptorchid epididymis is compared to its descended partner the following morphological differences are apparent (Fig. 16):

1. the whole epididymis is shorter and has fewer coils;
2. the interstitium of the cryptorchid epididymis is broader with an extensive mesenchymal condensation around the tubulus cross-section;
3. the head and tail of this epididymis are less developed;
4. the head of epididymis is dissociated from the apex of the testis (Fig. 17).

The underdeveloped epididymis is also encountered in adult cryptorchid patients [40]. Its interstitium is even wider than that of a cryptorchid boy and the ductus epididymidis atrophy is more prominent [40]. Compared to the normal descended epididymis of adult males it is evident that the whole ductus is shorter. This indicates that after puberty permanent impairment of the epididymis development and differentiation exists, although normal plasma testosterone and "normalization" of the partial gonadotropin deficiency is achieved.

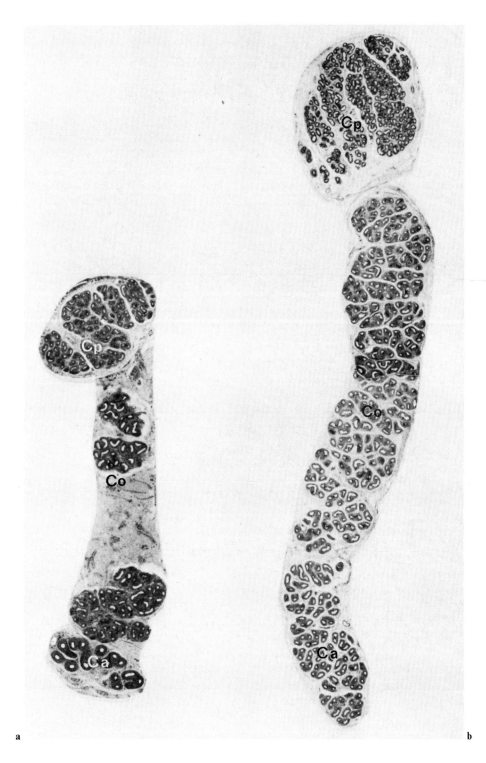

a   b

Fig. 16. Photomontage of a cryptorchid (**a**) and a descended (**b**) epididymis in an unilateral cryptorchid full-term newborn. The cryptorchid epididymis is shorter, displaying fewer tubules and an underdeveloped caput (*Cp*), corpus (*Co*) and cauda (*Ca*). Cryptorchid testis was located intraabdominally. (14×)

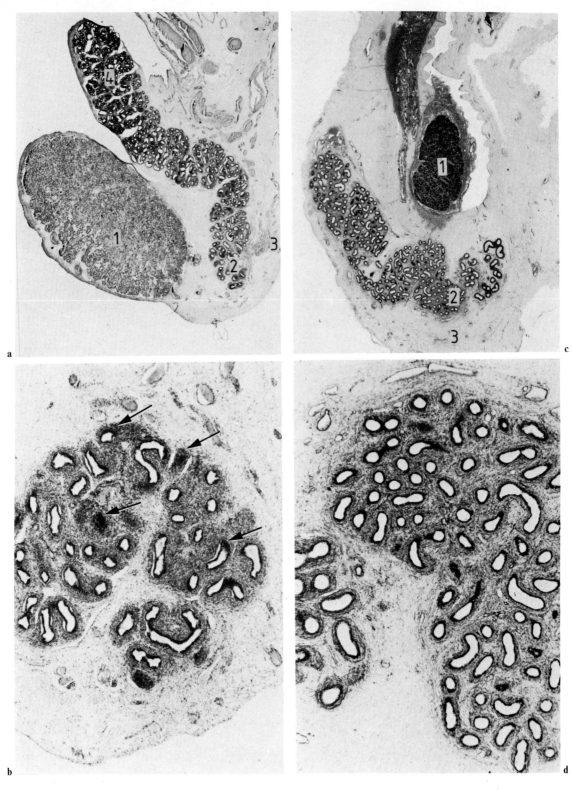

Fig. 17. a Cryptorchid epididymis of a newborn showing a dissociation between the head (*4*) of the epididymis and the testis (*1*). The cauda epididymidis (*2*) is underdeveloped when compared to the cauda epididymidis of a normally descended testis. (*3*) gubernaculum. **b** Histological section of cryptorchid cauda epididymidis possessing fewer tubules and a strong condensation of mesenchymal tissue around it (*arrow*). **c, d** Histological section through the cauda epididymidis of a normally descended testis. No mesenchymal condensations (as in **b**) are discernible and abundancy of the tubules is evident

References

1. Falin IL (1969) The development of genital glands and the origin of germ cells in human embryogenesis. Acta Anat 72:195–232
2. Peters H (1976) Intrauterine gonadal development. Fertil Steril 27:493–499
3. Jirasek EJ (1970) The relationship between differentiation of the testicle, genital ducts and external genitalia in fetal and postnatal life. In: Rosenberg E, Paulsen CA (eds) The human testis. Plenum Press, New York London
4. Ohno S, Nagai Y, Ciccarese S, Iwata H (1979) Testis organizing H-Y antigen and the primary sex-determining mechanism of mammals. Recent Prog Horm Res 35:449
5. Wachtel SS, New IM (1981) Studies on H-Y antigen: The genetic basis of abnormal gonadal differentiation. In: Kogan SJ, Hafez ESE (eds) Pediatric andrology. Martinus Nijhoff, The Hague, Boston London
6. Wolf U (1979) XY gonadal dysgenesis and the H-Y antigen. Human Genet 47:269–277
7. Stieve H (1930) Männliche Genitalorgane. In: Oksche A, Vollrath L (eds) Handbuch der mikroskopischen Anatomie der Menschen. Vol 7/2 Springer, Berlin
8. Fischel A (1930) Über die Entwicklung der Keimdrüsen des Menschen. Z Anat Entwicklungsgesch 92:34–72
9. Witschi E (1951) Embryogenesis of the adrenal and the reproductive gland. Recent Prog Horm Res 6:1–27
10. Witschi E (1956) Developments of vertebrates. Saunders, Philadelphia
11. Wartenberg H (1978) Human testicular development and the role of the mesonephros in the origin of a dual Sertoli cell system. Andrologia 10:1–21
12. Gipouloux J-D (1962) Les tissus mésodermiques dorsaux exercent-ils une action attractive sur les gonocytes primordiaux situés dans l'endoderme chez l'embryon du crapaud commun Bufo bufo L. (Amphibien anoure)? CR Acad Sci (Paris) 255 (11):2179–2181
13. Fukuda T, Hedinger Chr, Groscurth P (1975) Ultrastructure of developing germ cells in the fetal human testis. Cell Tiss Res 161:55–70
14. Fukuda T (1976) Ultrastructure of primordial germ cells in human embryo. Virchows Archiv [Cell Pathol] 20:85–89
15. Hadžiselimović F (1976) Elektronsko mikrokopska proučavanja promjena na gonocitima djece neposredno poslije rodjenja. Folia Anat Jugos 5:37–43
16. Seguchi A, Hadžiselimović F (1974) Ultramikroskopische Untersuchungen am Tubulus seminiferous bei Kindern von der Geburt bis zur Pubertät. I. Spermatogonienentwicklung. Verh Anat Ges 68:133–148
17. Hadžiselimović F (1977) Cryptorchidism. Adv Anat Embryol Cell Biol 53/3
18. Hilscher W (1974) Kinetik der Präspermatogenese und Spermatogenese. Verh Anat Ges 68:39–62
19. Holstein AF, Wartenberg H, Vossmeyer J (1971) Zur Cytologie der pränatalen Gonadenentwicklung beim Menschen. III. Die Entwicklung der Leydig-Zellen im Hoden von Embryonen und Feten. Z Anat Entwicklungsgesch 135:43–46
20. Lameh NC (1960) A study of the development and structural relationships of the testis and gubernaculum. Surg Gynecol Obstet 110:164–192
21. Jost A (1946/47) Recherches sur la différenciation sexuelle de l'embryon de lapin. I. Introduction et embryologie génitale normale. II. Action des androgènes de synthèse sur l'histogenèse génitale. III. Rôle des gonades foetales dans la différenciation sexuelle somatique. Arch Anat Microsc Morphol Exp 36:151–200; 242–270; 271–315
22. Backhouse MK (1981) Embryology of the normal and cryptorchid testis. In: Fonkalsrud WE, Mengel W (eds) The undescended testis. Year Book med cal Publishers, Chicago London
23. Hollinshead WH (1971) Anatomy for surgeons, vol 2. The thorax, abdomen and pelvis. Harper and Row, New York Evanston San Francisco London
24. Van de Velde RL (1963) The origin and development of smooth muscle and contractility in the ductus epididymidis of the rat. J Embryol Exp Morphol 11:369–382
25. Cattenach BM, Iddon CA, Charlton HM, Chiappa SA, Fink L (1977) Gonadotropin-releasing hormone deficiency in a mutant mouse with hypogonadism. Nature 269:338–339
26. Green RR, Burill MW, Ivy AC (1938) Experimental intersexuality. The production of feminized male rats by antenatal treatment with estrogens. Science 88:130–131
27. Neumann F, Kramer M (1964) Antagonism of androgenic and antiandrogenic in their action on the rat fetus. Endocrinology 75:428–433
28. Elger W, Neumann F, Berswordt-Wallrabe R von (1971) The influence of androgen antagonists and progestagens on the sex differentiation of different mammalian species. In: Hainburgh H, Barrington EJW (eds) Hormones in development. Appleton-Century-Crofts. Educational Division. Mercolith Corporation, New York
29. Wensing CJG (1973) Testicular descent in some domestic mammals. III. Search for the factors that regulate the gubernacular reaction. Proc Kan Akad Wetensch C 76:196–200
30. Wensing CJG, Colenbrander B (1977) The process of normal and abnormal testicular descent. In: Bierich JR, Roger K, Ranke MB (eds) Maldescensus testis. Urban & Schwarzenberg, Baltimore Wien München
31. Hamilton JB (1938) The effect of male hormone upon the descent of the testis. Anat Res 70:533–541
32. Wells LJ (1943) Descent of the testis. Surgery 14:436–472
33. Raynaud A (1942) Modification expérimentale de la différenciation sexuelle des embryons des souris par action des hormones androgènes et oestrogènes. Paris, Herman
34. Donahoe KP, Ho Y, Morikawa Y, Hendren HW (1977) Müllerian Inhibiting Substance in human testis after birth. J Pediatr Surg 12:322–330
35. Donahoe KP, Budzik PG, Swenn AD (1981) The biochemistry and biology of Müllerian inhibiting substance. In: Kogan JS, Hafez ESE (eds) Pediatric andrology. Martinus Nijhoff, The Hague Boston London
36. Hadžiselimović F, Herzog B, Girard J (1976) Impaired intrauterine gonadotropin secretion as an etiological component of cryptorchidism. Pediatr Res 10:883
37. Hadžiselimović F, Herzog B, Seguchi J (1975) Surgical correction of cryptorchidism at 2 years. Electron microscopic and morphometric investigations. J Pediatr Surg 10:19–28

38. Hadžiselimović F, Girard J (1977) Pathogenesis of cryptorchidism. Hormone Res 8:76–83

39. Hadžiselimović F, Herzog B, Kruslin E (1978) The morphological background of estrogen-induced cryptorchidism in the mouse. Folia Anat Jugos 8:63–73

40. Hadžiselimović F, Girard J, Herzog B (1980) Die Bedeutung des Nebenhodens für den Descensus Testiculorum. Helv Paediat Acta Suppl 45:34

41. Rajfer J, Walsh CP (1977) Testicular descent. In: Blandau JR, Bergsma D (eds) Birth defects. Original Article Series Vol. 13, No. 2: Morphogenesis and malformation of the genital system. Liss, New York

42. Hadžiselimović F (1981) Funktionelle Morphologie und Pathologie der Nebenhoden und ihr Einfluß auf den Descensus testiculorum. Morphol Med 1:31–42

43. Barrow M, Gough MH (1970) Bilateral absence of testes. Lancet 1:366

44. Dickinson SJ (1973) Structural abnormalities in the undescended testis. J Pediatr Surg 8:523–527

45. Dean LA jr, Major WJ, Ottenheimer JE (1952) Failure of fusion of the testis and epididymis. J Urol 68:754–758

46. Lythgoe PJ (1961) Failure of fusion of the testis and epididymis. Br J Urol 33:80–85

47. Davis LE, Shpall AR, Goldstein BMA, Morrow WJ (1974) Congenitally uncoiled epididymis in a cryptorchid testicle. J Urol 111:618–620

48. Michelson L (1942) Congenital anomalies of the ductus deferens and epididymis. J Urol 61:389–390

49. Marshall FF, Shermeta WD (1979) Epididymal abnormalities associated with undescended testis. J Urol 121:341–343

50. Bramann F (1884) Beiträge zur Lehre vom Descensus testiculorum und dem Gubernaculum Hunteri beim Menschen. Müllers Archiv

51. Bramann F, 1914 cited by Müller A (1938) Individualität und Fortpflanzung als Polaritätserscheinung. Gustav Fischer, Jena, p 7

52. Michalek HL, Krepp J (1972) Failure of urogenital union with secondary amputation of the epididymal tail: a case report with complete review of literature. J Urol 107:436–439

53. Priesel A (1924) Über das Verhalten von Hoden und Nebenhoden bei angeborenem Fehlen des Ductus deferens. Virchows Arch [Pathol Anat] 249:246–304

54. Hanley HG, Hodges RD (1959) The epididymis in male sterility. A preliminary report of microdissection studies. J Urol 82:508–520

55. Scorer CG, Farrington GH (1980) Congenital abnormalities of the testis: Cryptorchidism, testicular torsion, and inguinal hernia and hydrocele. In: Harrison HJ, Gilles FR, Perlmutter DA, Stamey AT, Walsh CP (eds) Campbell's urology, 4th edn. Saunders, Philadelphia

4 Histology and Ultrastructure of Normal and Cryptorchid Testes

F. Hadžiselimović

4.1 Development of the Normal Testis in Children

4.1.1 First Year of Life [1]

Immediately after birth, the seminiferous tubule is composed of gonocytes, spermatogonia and Sertoli cells. The gonocytes or primitive reproductive cells are located mainly in the centre of the tubule and show a tendency to move towards the basement membrane. Two different types of gonocytes can be distinguished (Fig. 1, Chap. 3). When the gonocyte comes into contact with the basement membrane, it changes into a fetal spermatogonium, the largest cell in the infant seminiferous tubule (Fig. 1, Chap. 3). The most common cell in the seminiferous tubule in the 1st year is the Sertoli cell, an oval or polarized cell which, by definition, is always in contact with the basement membrane (Figs. 1, 2, 3a). It is a small cell (410 μ^3) fulfilling, in addition to phagocytizing, hormone-producing, and nutritive functions, a supporting role (Figs. 1, 2, 3a).

The peritubular connective tissue, which forms the wall of the seminiferous tubule, is composed of the basement membrane, here consisting of one layer, a collagen fiber zone and fibroblasts (Fig. 3b). The fibroblasts form concentric rings around the tubule. The interstitium contains mainly fetal Leydig cells, which are well developed and can be found in the interstitium until the 2nd year (Fig. 3b; see also Chap. 3).

4.1.2 Fourth Year [1]

The seminiferous tubule has an ultrastructural appearance quite different from that of a 1-year-old. Gonocytes are no longer visible. In addition to the A-type spermatogonia, which can already be seen in the 1-year-old, B-type spermatogonia are encountered for the first time (Fig. 4). Simultaneously with the appearance of B-type spermatogonia, primary spermatocytes are found in the seminiferous tubule. The Sertoli cells have completed their transformation from fetal cells into Sa- and Sb-type cells (Fig. 5). The Sa-type cell is the most common of the Sertoli cells in the seminiferous tubule in children. In the 4th year, simultaneously with the appearance of the B spermatogonia and primary spermatocytes, Sb-type Sertoli cells are found in increasing numbers (Fig. 5).

Apart from a certain widening, there are no qualitative changes in the peritubular connective tissue. The basement membrane still consists of one layer and no knob formation is discernible. The collagen fiber layer is wider and the cellular layer is composed of fibroblasts. The interstitium contains mainly precursors of Leydig cells, but occasionally, however, particularly between the ages of 4 and 8 years, juvenile Leydig cells can be seen grouped around the vessels (Fig. 6a).

4.1.3 Puberty [1]

In puberty the final development of all four elements is completed. The Sertoli cells increase to as much as five times their previous size and the transition to the Sc-type cell takes place (Figs. 7, 3). The number of Sertoli cells has been steadily decreasing from birth to puberty. The seminiferous tubule acquires a lumen and degenerating cells are very seldom seen. The germ cells comprise spermatogonia, primary spermatocytes, secondary spermatocytes, and spermatids. Up until the age of 14 it was impossible to locate any sperm in our material. Only when the Sertoli cells are fully developed does the sperm appear. In the peritubular connective tissue a change takes place under the influence of gonadotropin. The basement membrane

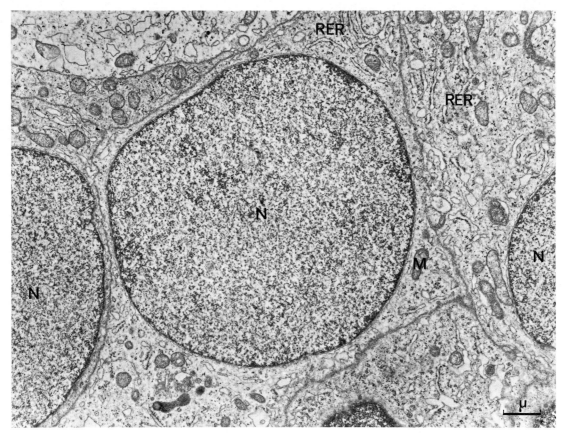

Fig. 1. Sa type Sertoli cell. The nucleus (*N*) is round with its chromatin finely dispersed. The narrow cytoplasm con-tains mitochondria (*M*) and rough endoplasmic reticulum (*RER*)

becomes multilayered and a knob formation becomes visible. The collagen fibers run in an orderly fashion and a transformation from fibroblasts to myofibroblasts takes place. The seminiferous tubule thus acquires a certain con-tractility (Fig. 8).

The Leydig cells are very well developed, with a particularly noticeable increase in the amount of smooth endoplasmic reticulum (Fig. 6b). However, no Reinecke's crystalloids are as yet visible. The morphometric analysis of 1- to 6-year-old testes compared to 13-year-old testes shows that the proportion of Sertoli cells de-creases from 91% to 72%. Furthermore, an in-crease of 14.5% in germ cells takes place, as well as an increase of 4.5% of degenerating cells (Fig. 9). The decrease in the number of Sertoli cells with increasing age corresponds favorably with the observation that after birth mitosis of these cells does not occur [1].

During childhood the Sertoli cells were small. The single cell volume was about 410 μ^3 in the 1st year of life and in the 12th year 1,500 μ^3. There was a sudden increase of single cell vol-ume in the 13th year of life (3,450 μ^3) which coincided with the enlargement of the diameter of the seminiferous tubule. In the first group (1st–6th year) the Sertoli cells were comprised of 28% nucleus and 72% cytoplasm. In the sec-ond group (10th–13th year) the percentage of cytoplasm increased to 81%, and that of the nucleus decreased to 19%. The volume density of Sertoli cell cytoplasm increased by 11% (ref-erence volume: Sertoli cell), but if the reference volume was testicular tissue, there was a 24% decrease of Sertoli cell cytoplasm. With the advance of puberty, the volume density of the Sertoli cells decreased by 33% (reference vol-ume: testicular tissue). In the first group, the number of Sertoli cell nuclei was 1,461 × 10⁶

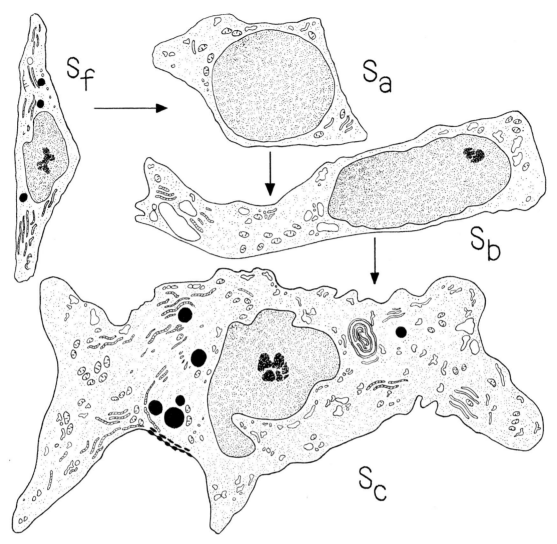

Fig. 2. Different types of Sertoli cells. The Sf fetal Sertoli cell is transformed after birth into the Sa type cell, which gives rise to the Sb type cell. In puberty, Sa and Sb cells transform into the Sc type due to increased gonadotropin and testosterone stimulation

(reference volume: testicular tissue), compared to 553×10^6 in the second group (reference volume: testicular tissue). This was a decrease of about 64%. The Sertoli cell cytoplasm in the first group consisted of 89% ground substance, 4% mitochondria, 5% Golgi apparatus, 1.2% vacuoles, and 0.8% lipoid droplets and lysosomes. In the second group, 82.4% was ground substance, 7.6% mitochondria, 3.6% Golgi apparatus, 2.2% vacuoles, and 4.1% lipoid droplets and lysosomes. The number of mitochondria rose from 200/Sertoli cell in the first group to 610/Sertoli cell in the second group, an increase of about 77%. At the same time, the absolute volume of mitochondria increased by 82% and there was an increase of 52% in the volume density of mitochondria (reference volume: Sertoli cell cytoplasm).

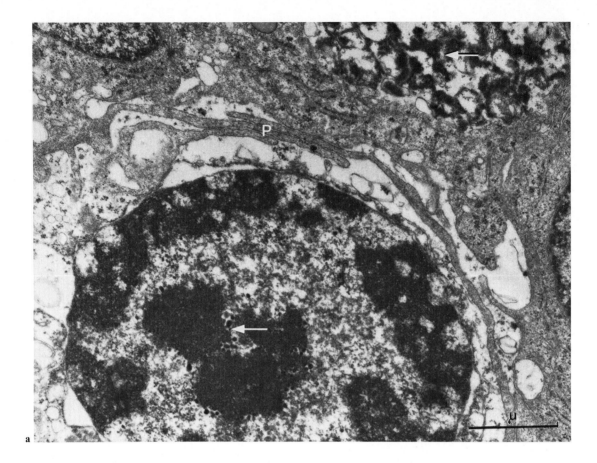

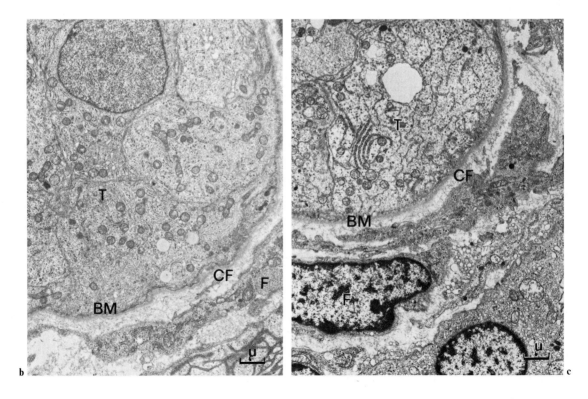

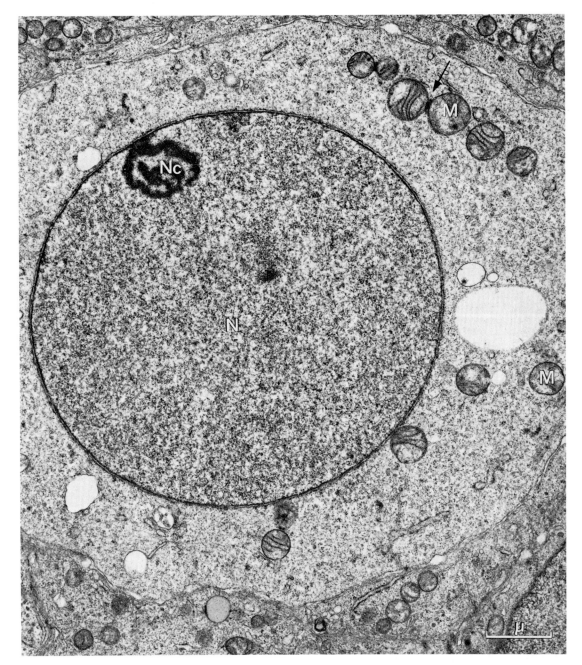

Fig. 4. Type B spermatogonia for the first time encountered in seminiferous tubule with a chronological age of 4 years. The mitochondria of crista type (*M*) very seldom have inter- mitochondrial cement (*arrow*), but are frequently dispersed singly throughout the whole electron-dense cytoplasm. The nucleolus (*Nc*) is peripherally situated in a round nucleus (*N*)

Fig. 3. a The phagocytosis of germ cells. The Sertoli cells enclose the degenerated gonocyte (↑) with their cytoplasmic processes (*P*). **b** Peritubular connective tissue of the semini- ferous tubule (*T*) of cryptorchid and normally descended (**c**) infant gonads. The collagen fiber layer (*CF*) appears identical in both testes. Fibroblast (*F*) is the outermost layer while the basement membrane (*BM*) is the innermost layer of the peritubular connective tissue

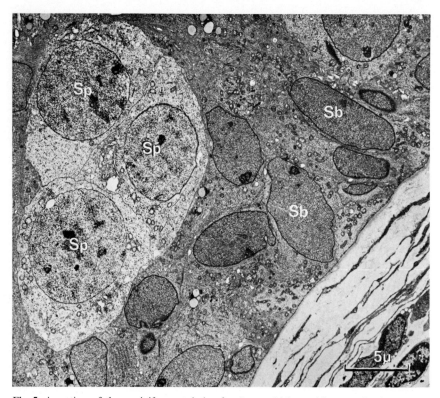

Fig. 5. A section of the seminiferous tubule of a 5-year-old boy with normally descended testis showing spermatocytes order I (*Sp*) and Sb type Sertoli cells (*Sb*)

Fig. 6. a Juvenile Leydig cells of a 6-year-old boy with normally descended testis. The nucleus (*N*) is irregular and its chromatin is condensed at its periphery. The nucleus displays large peripherally located nucleoli (*Nc*). In the narrow cytoplasm the main feature is a smooth endoplasmic reticulum (*SER*). **b** Details of the cytoplasm of a 13-year-old boy with descended testis. The increase in the amount of the smooth endoplasmic reticulum (*SER*) is apparent

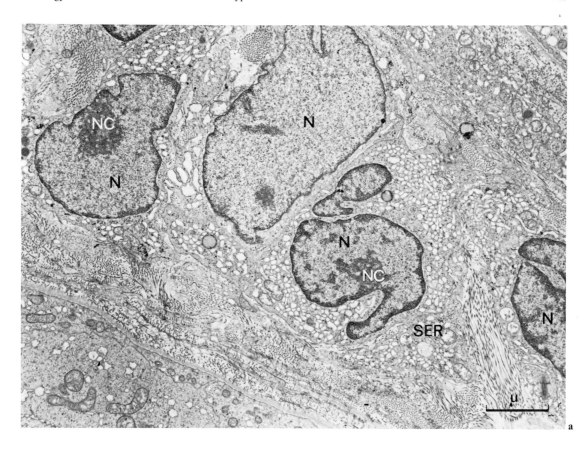

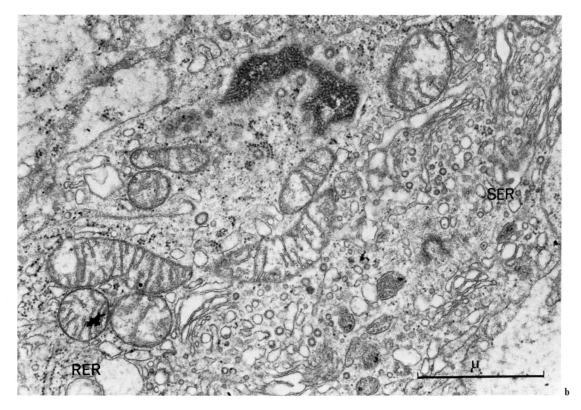

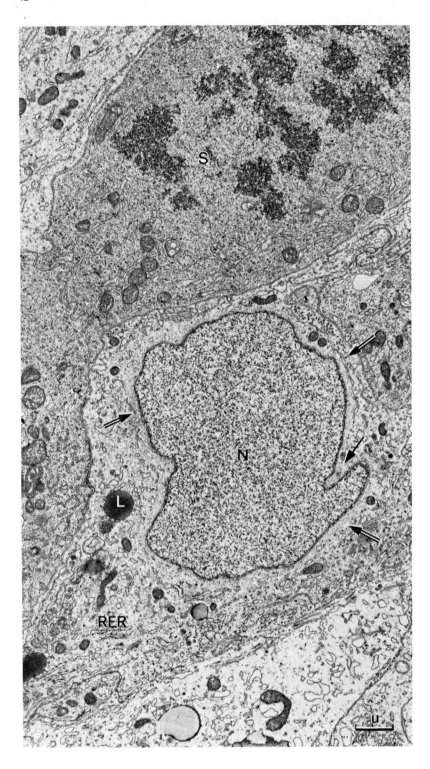

Fig. 7. Sc type Sertoli cell with a typical nucleus (*N*) displaying one or more deep invaginations (*arrow*). Around the nucleus a cytoplasmic "halo" is observable (*double arrows*). Lipoid droplets (*L*) and rough endoplasmic reticulum (*RER*) are scattered throughout the entire cytoplasm. In the vicinity a dividing spermatogonium (*S*) is observable

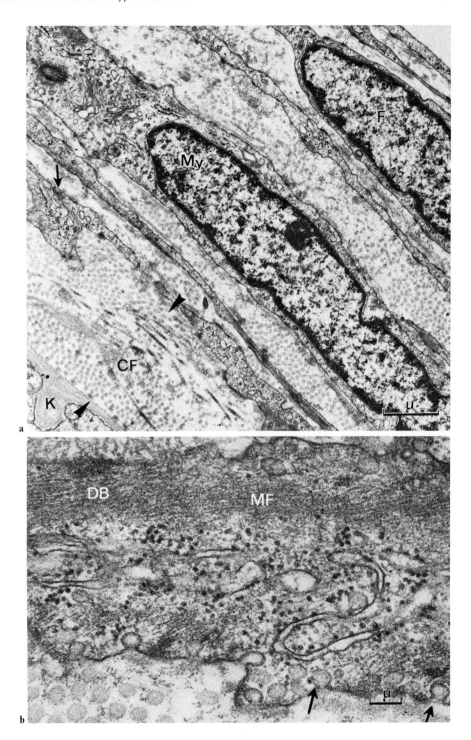

Fig. 8. a Peritubular connective tissue of a 13-year-old boy with normally descended testis. The multilayered basement membrane shows a knob-like structure (*K*). At least two different courses of collagen fibers within the collagen fiber layer (*CF*) are observable. The myofibroblasts are connected together over the gap junction (*My*). The fibroblasts (*F*) which are expected to create the Leydig cells are situated deeper in the interstitium. **b** Section of the cytoplasm of the myofibroblast with dense bodies (*DB*) and myofibrils (*MF*). Micropinocytosis is frequently observable at the cell surface (*arrow*)

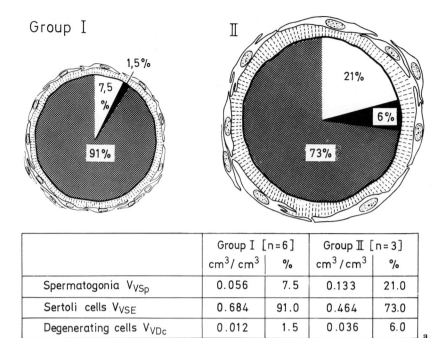

	Group I [n=6]		Group II [n=3]	
	cm^3/cm^3	%	cm^3/cm^3	%
Spermatogonia V_{VSp}	0.056	7.5	0.133	21.0
Sertoli cells V_{VSE}	0.684	91.0	0.464	73.0
Degenerating cells V_{VDc}	0.012	1.5	0.036	6.0

a

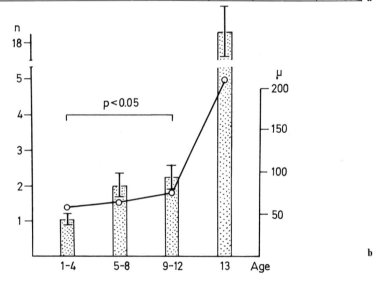

b

Fig. 9. a Morphometric analyses of the volume percentage of the distribution of three different cell types within the seminiferous tubule in the first 6 years of life in a normally descended testis (*I*) vs. early pubertal testis (*II*). The increase in volume of spermatogonia at the beginning of puberty is significant. **b** Development of the diameter of the semini-ferous tubule and the spermatogonia count per tubule cross section throughout childhood

4.2 Development of the Cryptorchid Testis

That the gonads in cryptorchid males have impaired reproductive function was stated by Hunter as early as 1785: "When one or both testicles remain through life in the belly, I believe they are exceedingly imperfect, and that this imperfection prevents the disposition for descent taking place" [2]. In the past 200 years several researchers attempted to prove the veracity of this statement. The most extreme proponents of the theory that a cryptorchid testis is congenitally malformed completely ignored any surgical effort to preserve a retained or partially descended testis, and considered this as something to be performed mainly for cosmetic reasons [3, 4]. However, Cooper noted in 1929 that the younger the age at which an undescended testis was examined histologically, the more closely the appearance approximated to normal. She also stated that the further the preadolescent testis had descended in its normal route, the more closely it corresponded histologically to the scrotal testis of the same age [5]. Obviously, the best method of resolving this controversy is to examine the whole development of cryptorchid and normal testes from birth until puberty is reached on an annual basis. During the past 10 years we have examined 721 cryptorchid testes varying from term newborns to adulthood. The development of normally descended testes was studied by light and electron microscope in 62 cases.

Even at a very low magnification the picture of a cryptorchid gonad is recognisable microscopically. A broad empty interstitium on the one hand and small tubules with a reduced number of germ cells on the other hand are typical features of prepubertal cryptorchid testes. Two peculiarities, namely circular tubules with spherical bodies and secondary areas of totally degenerated tubules are frequently observed within the undescended gonad.

The volume of tubules in a cryptorchid and scrotal gonad in prepubertal boys displays a retarded development throughout the whole childhood [6]. Not only is the amount of interstitial tissue impaired, but also the tubulus diameter in the testes of cryptorchid children is underdeveloped. However, the undescended testes in the first 5 years of life still have their tubule diameter within 2 SD of the norm [7, 8].

From infancy to puberty the total length of the seminiferous tubules increases from 100 m to 300 m [6]. This development is a continuous process throughout childhood. In a cryptorchid testis a severely impaired development of the length of the tubules has been identified; at the end of puberty the tubules are no longer than 100 m. In contrast, the tubules of the scrotal testis in unilateral cryptorchid boys reach, at the termination of puberty, the same length as those of a normally descended gonad (313.8 m ± 31 m) [6].

4.2.1 Behavior of the Number of Spermatogonia in Cryptorchid Gonads

4.2.1.1 In Relation to Age

In a normally descended gonad the number of spermatogonia increases continuously throughout childhood. After puberty the testis has approximately 800,000,000 spermatogonia [6]. It is important to stress that within the first 6 months of life all cryptorchid testes had germ cells within the norm. This is based on the published reports detailing 78 cases [9–20] and our own observation of 32 cases. As early as the 2nd year of life 22% of cryptorchid testes in unilateral cryptorchid boys had completely lost their germ cells. The development of the germ cells in a cryptorchid gonad from the 2nd year of life was severely inhibited (Fig. 10). The mean number of spermatogonia per tubule remained from the 2nd year until puberty ∼ 0.38 constant (Fig. 11). The scrotal gonad in unilateral cryptorchidism had as a rule more germ cells than the cryptorchid gonad, but sig-

Table 1. Morphometry of the tubulus seminiferous in normal and cryptorchid prepubertal testis

Morphometrical symbol	Normal testis		Cryptorchid testis	
	Mean	S.E.	Mean	S.E.
Number of Sertoli cell nuclei/cm^3	1,461 $\times 10^6$	134 $\times 10^6$	1,17 $\times 10^6$	103 $\times 10^6$
Single cell volume/μ^3	491	55	429	17
Volume density of spermatogonia/cm^3	0056	0018	0021	0009
Volume density of degenerating cells	0012	0003	0018	0006

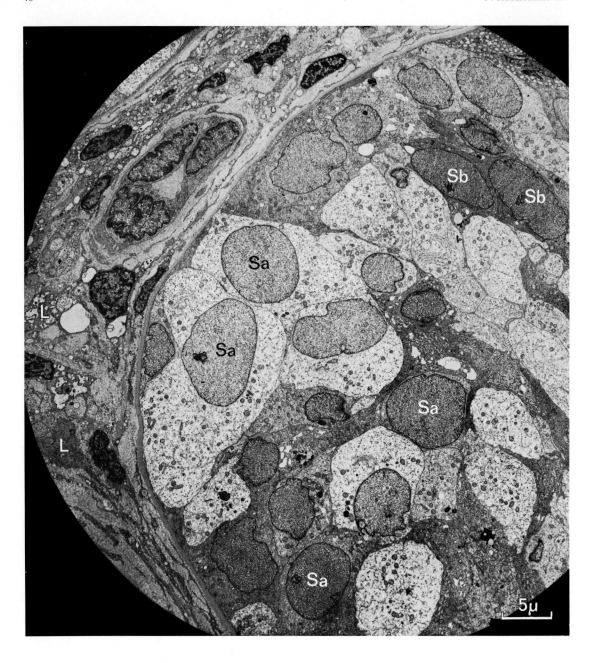

Fig. 10. The seminiferous tubule of a 4-year-old cryptorchid boy, encountering only Sertoli cells of Sa and Sb type. The different appearance of the cytoplasm of these cells (pale/ dark) is to be interpreted as being due to different functional stages. Within the interstitium the atrophic Leydig cells (*L*) are present

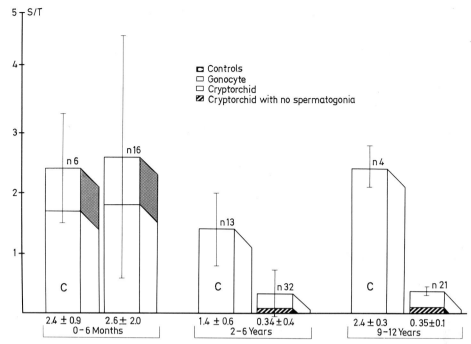

Fig. 11. Spermatogonia count (*S/T*) per seminiferous tubule cross section in cryptorchid and normally descended testes of various ages

nificantly less than a normally descended gonad of a similar age (Fig. 12). The volume density of the spermatogonia in 1- to 6-year-old cryptorchid boys was examined morphometrically and was found to amount to 0.056 cm^3 testicular tissue in the control testes and 0.021 spermatogonia/cm^3 testicular tissue in the cryptorchid testes, which is equivalent to a decrease in volume density of spermatogonia of approximately 60%. The difference between these two groups is thus significant ($P < 0.005$) (Table 1) [1].

4.2.1.2 In Relation to Position

The TFI (tubule fertility index) depends on the position at which the testis is retained. The mean TFI (percentage of testicular tubules seeming to contain spermatogonia) of intra-abdominal testes (4.8%) is significantly less than that of testes retained in the inguinal canal (19.1%) ($P < 0.005$) [11]. This in turn is less than the TFI of the testes in the superficial inguinal pouch (31.4%), which themselves have a lower TFI than do those testes arrested high in the scrotum (42.4%) [11]. However, on spermatogonia count per 50 tubule cross section there is a significant difference only between

intra-abdominally and suprascrotally located testes (Table 2). It should be noted that all intra-abdominal testes do have germ cells with-

Table 2. Spermatogonia count per tubule (S/T) with regards to the position of the testis

	I Abdominal		II Inguinal		III Suprascrotal	
	S/T	Age (years)	S/T	Age (years)	S/T	Age (years)
1	0.0	11.0	0.0	6.1	0.0	4.8
2	0.0	10.5	0.0	6.9	0.0	4.8
3	0.0	4.8	0.34	6.6	0.93	8.11
4	0.0	3.1	0.0	11.3	1.60	7.8
5	0.0	8.11	0.0	3.6	2.40	7.8
6	0.16	5.0	0.7	4.4	0.63	6.3
7			0.0	5.8	1.22	4.5
8			0.21	5.9	0.08	3
9			0.46	6.7	0.23	10.5
10			0.90	10.8	0.16	3
11			0.21	11.3		
12			0.38	5.9		
Mean		7.3		7.1		6.0
±SD		±3		±2.6		±2.4

I:III   2 α < 0.05 Wilcoxon test
I:II   }
II:III }   n.s.

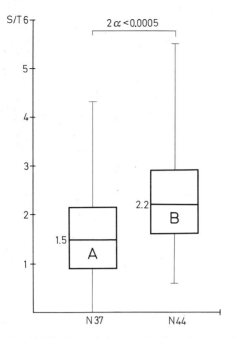

Fig. 12. The descended testes of unilateral cryptorchid boys are compared according to the spermatogonia count in their cryptorchid gonads. Group A had no germ cells in the cryptorchid gonad and a significantly lower spermatogonia count in the descended gonads than group B. The latter group had a spermatogonia/tubules count (S/T) of >0.5 in cryptorchid gonads. The *line* within the bar represents median values for S/T, the *bar* represent the interquartile range. The *vertical lines* give the whole range (Wilcoxon test was performed). The data from ref. (6, 19) together with our data were used

in the first 6 months of life. After this period, the most significant loss of germ cells during childhood occurred in the intra-abdominal testes. Six of seven prepubertal intra-abdominal testes had a complete lack of germ cells (91%). In inguinally located testes 41% had no germ cells, while in prescrotal testes the total absence of germ cells was noted in only 20% of the patients. The superficial ectopic testes (obstructed) had the same mean number of spermatogonia as the prescrotal ones, indicating that this type of "ectopic" testis had the same degree of testicular tissue damage (Table 2).

4.2.2 Ultrastructure of Cryptorchid Testis

4.2.2.1 Germ Cells

In the 1st year, in addition to the fetal spermatogonia, gonocytes are also occasionally present in the seminiferous tubule of cryptorchid infants. The fetal spermatogonia are ultrastructurally identical to those in normal testes in children of the same age. Rarely, transitional and Ap and Ad spermatogonia can also be observed. The Ap, Ad, and transitional spermatogonia appear to be fewer in number than in the normal control testes [1], but have the same ultrastructure as in normal testes (Fig. 13a).

By the age of 3 years, the qualitative changes in the spermatogonia of cryptorchid testes have become marked. Bi-nuclear spermatogonia are encountered more frequently than in normal testes (Fig. 13b). The spermatogonia are mostly fetal or of transient type, sometimes with bizarre nuclear structures. The mitochondria of these fetal spermatogonia, which are reduced in number, are of the crista and tubule type. In contrast to normal spermatogonia, they have an increased number of large, membrane-bounded vacuoles, with inhomogeneously distributed contents [1]. These could be phagocytized cell elements, although no active spermatogonia phagocytosis was observed. Histometric comparison of the spermatogonia of 3-year-old and 1-year-old cryptorchids shows a considerable alteration in the nucleus-plasma ratio in favour of the nucleus [21], the cytoplasm of most spermatogonia appearing electron-darker than normal spermatogonia of the same age. The Golgi apparatus and the endoplasmic reticulum show scarcely any development.

The marked reduction in spermatogonia in the 6-year-old is obvious for fetal, transitional and Ap spermatogonia; Ad spermatogonia are rarely seen and primary spermatocytes are never observed. All the forms of spermatogonia have a narrower cytoplasm, which appears electron-darker than that of the control spermatogonia and becomes increasingly reduced with

Fig. 13. a Three-nuclear transient type spermatogonia within the seminiferous tubule of a 10-year-old boy. A typical perinucleolar halo is evident (*arrow*). **b** Ap spermatogonia in a 10-year-old cryptorchid boy (S). The nucleus (N) has a peripherally located nucleolus (*Nc*). The mitochondria (*M*) are connected with intermitochondrial cement (*arrows*). The Sertoli cells are of the Sa type (*Sa*)

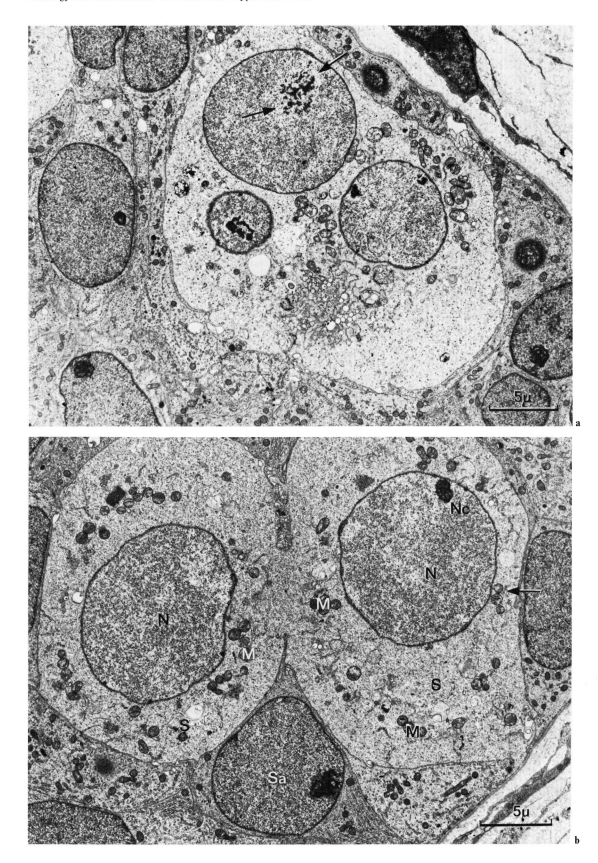

age. The eccentrically situated nucleus has a loose, reticular, well-developed nucleolus, with round mitochondria which vary greatly in size. Large, membrane-bounded vacuoles, sometimes in contact with mitochondria, are also frequently present in the cytoplasm of all types of spermatogonia. The Golgi apparatus and endoplasmic reticulum are poorly developed [1]. The majority of the spermatogonia show signs of incipient degeneration [1]. All stages of transition up to the complete degeneration of the cell can be observed [1].

4.2.2.2 Sertoli Cells [1]

In cryptorchid testes too, the cells most frequently encountered in the seminiferous tubule are the Sertoli cells. On the basis of their morphology, two types can be distinguished before puberty, namely the Sa type and the Sb type. The fetal Sertoli cells, which in normal testes persist until the 3rd month post natum, were almost nonexistent in our material as early as 2 weeks after birth, the Sa-type Sertoli cells occupying the greater part of the seminiferous tubule. The Sa type, with its large, round nucleus and only slightly differentiated cytoplasm, shows hardly any qualitative differences from the Sa type cell of normal testes until puberty. The Sb type, on the other hand, is much rarer and the isolated cells seem to have less smooth endoplasmic reticulum and lipoid droplets than those in normal testes from the same age group.

Morphometric assessment of the Sertoli cells up to the age of 6 years revealed no significant difference in number or in individual cell volume. The number of Sertoli cells per cubic centimeter testicular tissue in normal control testes was $1.441 \, cm^3 \times 10^6$, while in cryptorchid testes the figure was $1.617 \, cm^3 \times 10^6$, while in cryptorchid testes the figure was $1.617 \, cm^3 \times 10^6$. The single cell volume in normal testes is 491 μ^3 and in undescended testes 429 μ^3. The differences in the number of Sertoli cells and in single cell volume are not significant (Table 1).

In puberty, the transformation of the Sertoli cells to the Sc type is only partially completed. In most of the biopsy specimens examined from boys in puberty or immediately post puberty, the Sertoli cells remained at the Sa stage. In particular, the nucleus retains its round form and few uncharacteristic cell organelles can be found in the entire cytoplasm (Fig. 14). No crystalloid of Charcot-Böttcher is present and

the lamellar body is only incompletely developed. The number of lipoid droplets is extremely reduced.

4.2.2.3 Peritubular Connective Tissue

De la Balze et al. [22] described the changes in the tunica propria of cryptorchid testes, with particular reference to the fibrotic changes to be found in puberty. The thicker the tubule wall, the more marked were the changes in the tubule, with a resulting decrease in spermatogonia and changes in the Sertoli cells. Sohval [9] and Mancini et al. [23], working with the light microscope, noticed changes in the tunica propria in cryptorchid testes only in puberty. Georgiev and Markov [24], on the other hand, noticed fibrosis of the tunica propria as early as the age of 6 years, while in 8-year-olds they observed atrophic changes in the germinal epithelium. Only after puberty does the fibrositic tunica propria become hyalinized [24].

Leeson [25] carried out electron-microscopic studies on cryptorchid individuals between the ages of 4 and 38 years. A total of 22 patients were examined. In none of the children in the prepubertal period was he able to establish any pathological changes at an ultrastructural level. From the age of 10 onwards in cryptorchid individuals, a progressive fibrosis of the peritubular connective tissue set in, accompanied by delayed maturation of the seminiferous tubule. This fibrosis, which became more marked in the third group (14- to 38-year-olds) is, in his opinion, of particular significance.

The 721 biopsies examined in this study, taken from boys up to 16 years of age, only partly confirm Leeson's findings.

The first changes in the peritubular connective tissue take place in the 2nd year, when the collagen fiber layer shows an increase in collagen fibers, although the layer itself is not yet wider than in normal control testes of the same age [1].

In 3-year-olds, the changes in the peritubular connective tissue are still more marked. The collagen fiber layer in 3-year-old cryptorchid testes is broader and more collagenized than in controls of the same age (Fig. 15). The fibers lie close together and their diameter appears greater than in normal testes. Collagenization and widening of the tunica propria increase with age in cryptorchid testes. The biggest differences in the width of the peritubular connec-

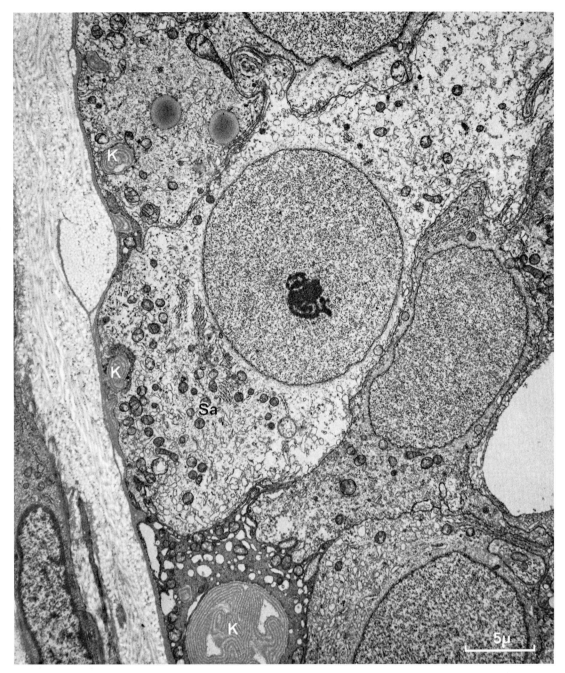

Fig. 14. Sa type Sertoli cells within the adult seminiferous tubule. This lack of transformation is frequently observable in adult cryptorchid testes. Basal membrane forms peculiar large knob formation (*K*)

tive tissue (i.e., the collagen fiber layer) between cryptorchid and normal testes are found in 7-year-olds. In fact the tunica propria continues to become wider with age in both cases, but the difference between them does not noticeably increase. The density of the collagen fibers and the fibrosis throughout the interstitium show a marked increase between the ages of 6 and 12, at which age the whole interstitium appears intensively collagenized, with large accumulation of dense collagen fibers lying between isolated Leydig cells. The basement membrane shows no differences compared with the normal testis until puberty, when the normal lamellari-

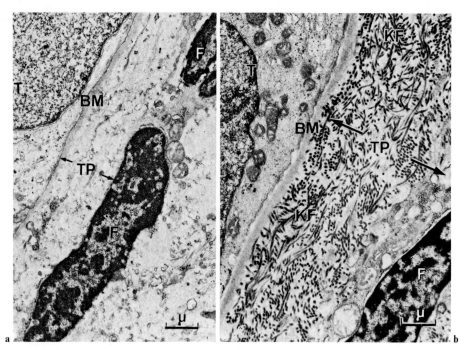

Fig. 15. Peritubular connective tissue in a 3-year-old cryptorchid boy (**b**) compared to a normally descended testis of the same age (**a**). The collagen fiber layer (*TP*) is broader, more irregular, and denser in cryptorchid boys. The basement membrane (*BM*) is also thicker in cryptorchid boys. (*F*) fibroblasts; (*T*) seminiferous tubule; (*KF*) collagen fibres

zation of the basement membrane does not occur. The otherwise well-developed knobs on the basement membrane appear only in rudimentary form, and in several tubules the basement membrane exhibits marked irregularities and invaginations.

In 14-year-old cryptorchid testes, the collagen fiber layer has become wider and the collagen fibers are not arranged in orderly fashion. The six to seven cellular layers around the seminiferous tubule are reduced to two or three. The ring of cells, which should entirely surround the tubule, is imperfectly formed, the cells being grouped together in clumps, their processes only partially developed and the transformation from fibroblasts to myofibroblasts incomplete. The faulty development of the myofibroblasts and the marked fibrosis of the peritubular connective tissue not only make the tubule incapable of contraction but it may also be assumed that the large mucopolysaccharide deposits induced by the fibrosis hinder the exchange of substances between the seminiferous tubule and the interstitium.

The pathological mechanism responsible for the thickening of the wall of the seminiferous tubule in cryptorchidism is unclear. Gonadotropin deficiency is suggested [26]. Nevertheless, Usadel et al. [27] found unmyelinated nerve fibers in the walls of the testicular tubules, which react positively to cholesterase. It is possible that this is a very active process of penetration. The function of these nerve fibers, which are observed only in cryptorchids, never in normal testes, remains unclear [27]. Possibly these unmyelinated nerve fibers are involved in some way in the thickening of the wall of the seminiferous tubule in cryptorchidism.

4.2.2.4 Leydig Cells

Hayashi and Harrison [28] reported that in cryptorchid testes no Leydig cells were visible immediately after birth, in contrast to normal control testes where Leydig cells could be demonstrated with histological techniques throughout the 1st year.

At the ultrastructural level, a progressive degeneration in cryptorchid testes, beginning at the age of 5 years, was described [29]. Also a decrease in the number of Leydig cells compared to normal testes [29] was observed.

Using the electron microscope, it was possible to confirm, to a certain extent, the observations of Hayashi and Harrison. Unlike them, however, we did find Leydig cells in cryptorchid testes in 1-year-olds, lying singly in the interstitium. Their cytoplasm is much narrower than in normal control Leydig cells from the same age group. The nucleus is oval, with a prominent nucleolus and peripherally situated nuclear chromatin. Occasionally, empty vacuoles were found in the interior of the nucleus (Fig. 16b). When the Leydig cells are markedly atrophic or degenerating, the nucleus is no longer oval but irregular in shape, with numerous invaginations (Fig. 16a). The cytoplasm of these atrophic Leydig cells generally possess few uncharacteristic cell organelles, and fewer mitochondria and lipoid droplets are seen. The smooth endoplasmic reticulum, a typical feature of a fully developed Leydig cell, is very scarce here, vacuoles being more commonly encountered in the cytoplasm of these cells. The degenerating Leydig cells often have only cytolysosomes in their cytoplasm. The atrophic Leydig cells in the cryptorchid testis described above are strongly reminiscent of the picture of simple atrophy. From the 1st year until puberty, Leydig cells are very seldom found in the interstitium. In puberty, a retarded development of the Leydig cells takes place. Hormonal treatment, even when unsuccessful, induces the development and differentiation of the Leydig cells. After treatment the ultrastructural appearance of these cells closely resembles those of juvenile Leydig cells in normally descended testes (Fig. 16c). This indicates that after adequate hormonal stimulation the Leydig cells are able to develop and differentiate and that these cells are not congenitally malformed.

Summarizing the results of histological investigations, it is obvious that the difference between bilateral and unilateral cryptorchidism, considering the quality of the testicular tissue, is of a quantitative nature only, not a qualitative one.

4.2.3 Congenital or Acquired Lesions? Iatrogenic Cryptorchidism

The histological criteria for the congenital testicular defect is based upon two principal considerations: first, the verified absence of cytological components such as spermatogonia, Sertoli or Leydig cells unattributable to age, cryptorchidism, or postnatal factors [13]; and second, the persistence beyond the prepubertal era of immature seminiferous tubules [13].

The fact that 110 cryptorchid testes during the first 6 months of life had a normal number and appearance of germ, and Sertoli cells speaks undoubtedly against primary congenital testis malformation. Specifically it spoke against the hypothesis which interpreted the inability of the germ cells to divide as being due to a congenital malformation [11].

This stated inability of the spermatogonia in cryptorchid boys to undergo maturation themselves or to give rise to other cells capable of maturation is clearly rebutted by the observations of Bergada and Mancini [30]. They found that after HCG treatment of cryptorchid boys particularly the scrotal testis, in unilateral cryptorchid boys, reacts with significant histological changes, represented by an increase of the tubular diameter and proliferations of the germinal epithelium [30]. This was achieved after weekly injections of 1,000 U HCG for 3–6 months [30].

The poor response of the cryptorchid gonad observed during treatment is due to at least two factors: First, treatment was given when the gonad was still in a cryptorchid position and this could be inhibitory, as experiments on dogs showed [31]. Second, the youngest boy treated was 6 years old, at the time when 22% of the unilateral cryptorchid gonads already lack germ cells completely. That in these cases the response to the treatment was poor is not surprising.

In its most extreme expression anencephaly is characterized by a marked reduction of Leydig tissue (if not complete absence) while the tubules themselves appear superficially to be similar to those in controls, although the number of gonocytes in cross sections of the tubules appears to be much lower than in controls of the same age [32]. In other anencephalic fetuses damage to the testis was less severe. Some specimens contained a few Leydig cells and a seemingly normal population of gonocytes [32], while others possessed areas of intertubular connective tissue where in controls islands of Leydig tissue would normally be encountered [32]. The extent of the lesion within the fetal testis appeared to be related either to the extent of damage in the hypothalamus or

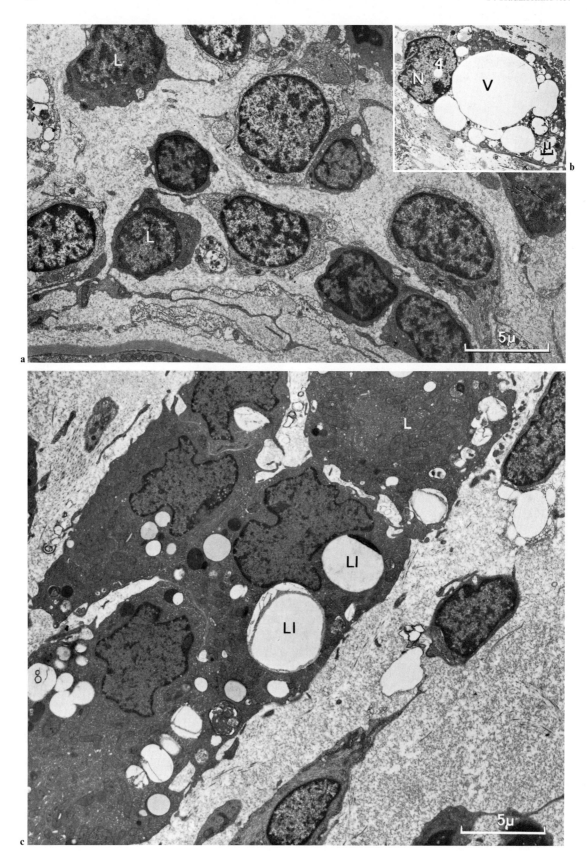

to the time when this damage became manifest. This histological picture closely resembles that of cryptorchid testes, specifically in the appearance of interstitial Leydig, and germ cells. There is a close relation between the severity of testicular damage and the impairment of the hypothalamo-pituitary-gonadal axis in cryptorchid boys. Furthermore, cryptorchidism appears frequently in anencephalic fetuses and is present in 44% of boys with cerebral lesions [33]. Not only a cryptorchid gonad in boys with hypothalamic lesions shows retarded development; also in a descended gonad a disturbance in the development was observed [34]. The partial isolated gonadotropin deficiency occurring in cryptorchid boys stops the transformation from A to B spermatogonia, as well as influencing to a certain extent multiplication of the germ cells. This is apparent if a congenitally cryptorchid gonad is compared to an iatrogenic cryptorchid gonad. Iatrogenic cryptorchidism resulting from hernia repair is one of the known complications [35]. The incidence given in the literature is less than 1% (2/237 children [35]). In the last 10 years we had nine cases of iatrogenic cryptorchidism after hernia repair. All children were infants when operated on and there was no particular predilection for one side or the other. The wound infections and testicular retractility appear to be factors predisposing this complication [35]. Although the iatrogenic cryptorchidism had the same maldescended position as the former one, even after 4 years of being in an unfavorable position, the transformation from A to B germ cells had occurred in these cryptorchid boys. The Leydig cells were normally developed in secondary cryptorchids until age 6 years and the interstitium was narrow (Fig. 17). However, the secondary changes due to an iatrogenically caused unfavorable position are observable: a diminution in the number of germ cells with big vacuoles within their cytoplasm and a thickening of the peritubular connective tissue (Fig. 17).

After 10 years of being in an unfavorable position, atrophic changes within the tubules are evident. The majority of the cells (Sertoli and spermatogonia) bear vacuoles in their cytoplasm and have pyknotic nuclei. The cell body of the spermatogonia is diminished (Fig. 17c).

4.2.4 Frequency and Ultrastructure of Carcinoma In Situ Cells in the Testes of Cryptorchid Children

It is generally assumed that the seminoma cells are derived from germinal cells. However, it is not known whether the tumor cells are abnormal germ cells that under unknown circumstances can, after puberty, undergo pathological proliferation, or whether they derive from adult spermatogonia [36]. In the latter case, spermatogonia should be influenced by an unknown factor. When more tumor cells were found within the tubule, fewer spermatogonia were observed. This observation lead to the hypothesis that intratubular seminoma cells are derived from spermatogonia [37]. To resolve this questionable thesis an examination of 721 cryptorchid testes was undertaken. In four testes intratubular seminoma cells were found. These cells closely resemble the primordial germ cells (Fig. 18). Their frequency is comparable to the frequency of carcinoma occurrence in the testis of cryptorchid patients. It may indicate that the intratubular seminoma cells are not transformed primordial germ cells dormant until puberty. It is also indicative that with the commencement of sperm production and increased hormonal stimulation of the testes they develop into seminoma.

The following are the similarities between primordial germ cells and carcinoma in situ cells:

1. The appearance of pseudopodia of various sizes extended from the cytoplasm
2. A pale nucleus with a centrally located prominent nucleolus
3. Huge aggregates of glycogen particles and bundles of tonofilaments
4. A microfilament with a diameter of approximately 60 Å, resembling the contractile elements in the myofibroblasts of the lamina propria.

Fig. 16. Atrophic Leydig cells (*L*) in a 10-year-old cryptorchid boy (**a**) and a cryptorchid newborn (**b**). A narrow cytoplasm with large vacuoles (*V*) and a hole (4) in the nucleus (*N*) are often observable phenomena. After hormonal treatment (unsuccessful) a marked enlargement of Leydig cell cytoplasm with an increase in lipoid droplets (*LI*) content takes place (**c**). The Leydig cells are now identical in their ultrastructure to the juvenile Leydig cells in a normally descended testis

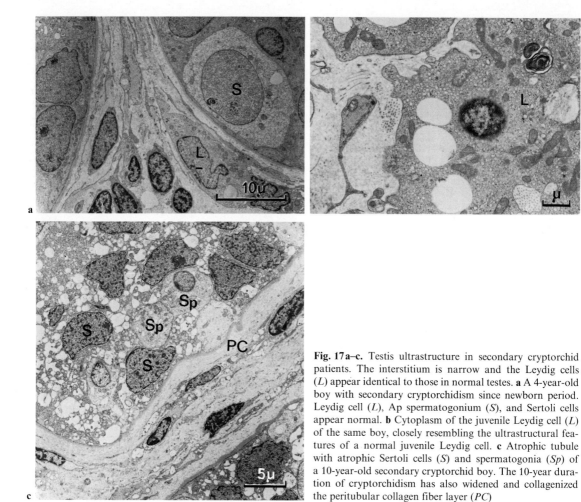

Fig. 17 a–c. Testis ultrastructure in secondary cryptorchid patients. The interstitium is narrow and the Leydig cells (*L*) appear identical to those in normal testes. **a** A 4-year-old boy with secondary cryptorchidism since newborn period. Leydig cell (*L*), Ap spermatogonium (*S*), and Sertoli cells appear normal. **b** Cytoplasm of the juvenile Leydig cell (*L*) of the same boy, closely resembling the ultrastructural features of a normal juvenile Leydig cell. **c** Atrophic tubule with atrophic Sertoli cells (*S*) and spermatogonia (*Sp*) of a 10-year-old secondary cryptorchid boy. The 10-year duration of cryptorchidism has also widened and collagenized the peritubular collagen fiber layer (*PC*)

Fig. 18. Carcinoma in situ cells in an adult male (**a**), a 12-year-old cryptorchid boy (**c**), and a 4-month-old cryptorchid infant (**b**). The typical features of these cells are their abundant storage of glycogen, a pale nucleus (*N*) with a large centrally located nucleolus (*Nc*), and a cytoplasm halo at the cell border (*arrow*). These cells, particularly those of the 4-month-old infant, resemble primordial germ cells. A lamellar body (*LB*) is also one of the characteristic structures

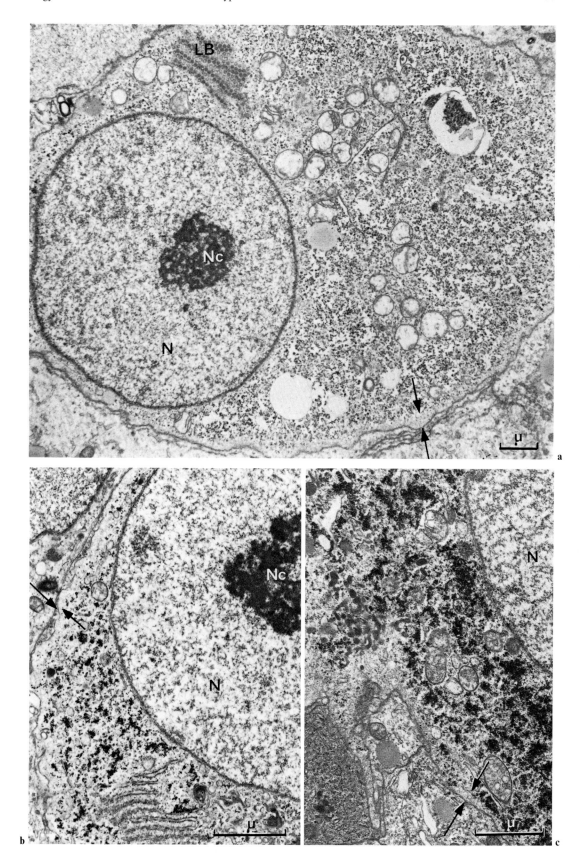

However, the appearance of lamellar bodies and crista-type mitochondria in carcinoma in situ cells gives two differences between them and the primordial germ cells. This does not allow us to declare that carcinoma in situ cells are a completely new cell type; rather we can say that they are nontransformed primordial germ cells with some differences acquired during childhood.

References

1. Hadžiselimović F (1977) Cryptorchidism. Adv Anat Embryol Cell Biol 53/3
2. Palmer JF (1837) The works of John Hunter. F.R.S. vol 4, London, Longman
3. Bland-Sutton J (1910) The values of the undescended testis. Practitioner 84:19
4. Charny CW, Wolgin W (1957) Cryptorchidism. Paul B. Hoeber, New York
5. Cooper ERA (1929) The histology of the retained testis in the human subject at different ages and its comparison with the scrotal testis. J Anat 64:5–27
6. Kleinteich B, Hadžiselimović F, Hesse V, Schreiber G (1979) Kongenitale Hodendystopien. VEB Georg Thieme, Leipzig
7. Hadžiselimović F (1981) Pathogenesis of cryptorchidism. In: Kogan SJ, Hafez ESE (eds) Pediatric andrology. Martinus Nijhoff, Den Hague
8. Bar-Maor JA, Nissan S, Lernau DZ, Oren M, Levy E (1979) Orchidopexy in cryptorchidism assessed by clinical, histologic and sperm examinations. Surg Gynecol Obstet 148:855–859
9. Sohval RA (1954) Histopathology of Cryptorchidism. Am J Med 16:346–362
10. Hösli PO (1971) Zur Problematik der Behandlung des Kryptorchismus. Aktuel Urol 2:107–120
11. Scorer CG, Farrington HG (1971) Congenital deformities of the testis and epididymis. Butterworths, London
12. Hecker WCh, Hienz HA, Mengel W (1972) Frühbehandlung des Maldenscensus testis. Dtsch Med Wochenschr 97:1325–1329
13. Brandesky G, Regele H (1973) Histologische Untersuchungen beim Leistenhoden. Monatsschr Kinderheilkd 121:611–613
14. Jendricke K, Rager K, Schäfer E, Reisert I (1973) Vorläufige Ergebnisse klinischer, biochemischer und anatomischer Untersuchungen bei Maldescensus testis. Kinderheilkd 121:634–635
15. Dougall AJ, McLean N, Wilkinson AW (1974) Histology of the maldescended testis at operation. Lancet 1:771–774
16. Knecht H (1976) Tubulusstruktur und Keimzellverteilung in frühkindlichen kryptorchen und normalen Hoden. Beitr Pathol 159:249–270
17. Meyer JM, Goldschmidt PA, Sauvage P, Buck P (1977) Etude histologique et histométrique du testicule ectopique en fonction de l'âge. Incidences thérapeutiques. Ann Chirur Infant [Paris] 18:371–378
18. Reisert I, Steinhardt B, Flach A, Tonutti E (1977) Spermatogonienzahl in descendierten und nicht descendier-
ten präpuberalen Hoden. Monatsschr Kinderheilkd 125:82–87
19. Hedinger Chr (1979) Histological data in cryptorchidism. In: Job JU (ed) Cryptorchidism. Pediatric Adolescent Endocrinology, Karger, Basel
20. Houissa S, Pape J de, Diebold N, Feingold J, Nezelof C (1979) Cryptorchidism. Histological study of 220 biopsies with clinico-anatomical correlations. In: Job JU (ed) Cryptorchidism, Pediatric Adolescent Endocrinology, Karger, Basel
21. Lüdin A (1977) Histometrische Untersuchungen an den Spermatogonien bei kryptorchen Knaben. Med. Dissertation Universität Basel
22. Balze de la FA, Mancini RE, Arrillaga F, Andrada JA, Vilar O, Gurtmann AI, Davidson OW (1960) Histologic study upon the undescended human testis during puberty. J Clin Endocrinol 20:286–297
23. Mancini ER, Rosenberg E, Cullen M, Lavieri CJ, Vilar O, Bergada C, Andrada AJ (1965) Cryptorchid and scrotal human testis. I. Cytological, cytochemical and quantitative studies. J Clin Endocrinol 25:927–942
24. Georgiev G, Markov D (1970) Histological changes in undescended testis. Sur Sci Med Verena 8:109–111
25. Leeson CR (1966) An electronmicroscopic study of cryptorchid and scrotal human testes, with special reference to pubertal maturation. Invest Urol 3:498–511
26. Bustos-Obregón E (1980) Peritubular tissue. In: Hafez ESE (ed) Descended and cryptorchid testis. Martinus Nijhoff, The Hague Boston London
27. Usadel HK, Schwedes U, Kollmann F, Dethe G (1977) Histological results of testis under normal conditions and in the development of primary hypogonadism in maldescensus testis. In: Maldescensus testis. Bierich RJ, Roger K, Ranke BM (eds) Urban & Schwarzenberg, München Wien Baltimore
28. Hayashi H, Harrison RG (1969) The development of the interstitial tissue of the human testis. Fertil & Steril 22:351–355
29. Numanoglu I, Köktürk I, Mutaf O (1969) Light and electronmicroscopic examinations of undescended testicles. J Pediatr Surg 4:614–619
30. Bergada C, Mancini ER (1973) Effect of gonadotropins in the induction of spermatogenesis in human prepubertal testis. J Clin Endocrinol Metab 37:935–943
31. Weissbach L, Heinemann I, Goslar GH (1975) Histochemische Untersuchungen beim experimentellen unilateralen Kryptorchismus des Hundes nach HCG-Behandlung. Acta Histochem 52:62–70
32. Baker GT, Scrimgeour BJ (1980) Development of the gonad in normal and anencephalic human fetuses. J Reprod Fertil 60:193–199
33. Ankerhold J, Gressmann C (1969) Hodendescensusstörungen beim frühkindlichen Hirnschaden. Z Kinderheilkd 107:15–25
34. Städtler F (1973) Die normale und gestörte präpubertale Hodenentwicklung des Menschen. Gustav Fischer, Stuttgart
35. Kaplan WG (1976) Iatrogenic cryptorchidism from hernia repair. Surg Gynecol Obstet 142:671–672
36. Holstein FA, Körner F (1974) Light and electron microscopical analysis of cell types in human seminoma. Virchows Arch [Pathol Anat] 363:97–112
37. Mostafi FK, Price BE (1973) Tumors of the male genital system. Armed Forces Institute of Pathology, Washington, D.C.

5 Endocrinology of the Hypothalamo-Pituitary-Gonadal Axis

F. Hadžiselimović

5.1 Development of the Hypothalamo-Pituitary-Gonadal Axis During Intrauterine Life in Normal Males

The hypothalamo-pituitary-gonadal axis controls testicular function and male reproduction. It begins to function in the prenatal period and undergoes continual development until puberty.

The positive immunoreactivity of the releasing hormone (GnRH) has been detected at around 4.5 weeks p.c. [1]. After 10 weeks, the pituitary LH and FSH are encountered [2]. The LH cells first appear in the pituitary and the gonadotropin concentrations increase rapidly, reaching their apex between the 20th and 25th week, and subsequently declining (Fig. 1) [2]. No significant sex differences concerning the serum level of fetal LH were observed [2].

The studies of pituitary endocrine function in four anencephalic infants showed that the response of FSH and LH was negative after the administration of 10 µg GnRH. On the contrary, no difference was found in plasma gonadotropins levels between anencephalic and normal infants [3]. The concentration of pituitary FSH and LH was significantly higher in female than in male fetuses, particularly from 15 to 29 weeks of gestation [2]. However, no correlation between pituitary content or concentration of LH or FSH and serum concentration of the retrospective hormone was found [2]. The sequential pattern of change in the concentration of both serum and pituitary LH and FSH is consistent with the development of a functional hypothalamo-pituitary-gonadal negative feedback system during fetal life [2].

The occurrence of hypotrophic genitalia and a reduced number of Leydig and germ cells in apituitary and anencephalic fetuses signify that pituitary LH may additionally influence the Leydig cell function and have a key function in promoting androgen secretion after genital differentiation is complete [4, 5, 6]. This interesting observation on apituitary and anencephalic fetuses, together with the experimental results of fetal hypophysectomy in rats and monkeys, has also shed new light on the role of FSH [6, 7]. The data obtained indicate that FSH is instrumental in the transformation of primordial germ cells into spermatogonia and may influence the differentiation of the Sertoli cells [6, 7].

The levels of HCG and testosterone in the male fetus are elevated during the critical period of Leydig cells and genital differentiation (8–12 weeks) [8]. The fetal HCG level parallels that of maternal serum, with peak levels between 17 and 19 weeks [3]. Its concentrations are on average 1/31 of those in maternal serum [8]. During the period of sexual differentiation, neither female nor male sex influences the maternal, fetal, or amniotic fluid HCG concentrations [8]. However, in the male fetus there is a definite correlation between HCG and testosterone [8]. In exclusive and outstanding work, Catt et al. established that fetal gonadotropins provided the hormonal stimulus for the maturation of the fetal Leydig cells and the onset of testosterone secretion [9]. The increase in the binding of gonadotropins in the fetal testis occurred precisely at the time when differentiation of the embryonic anlage was beginning [9].

5.2 Development of the Hypothalamo-Pituitary-Gonadal Axis in Normal Boys

At term and after birth the mean testosterone plasma level is higher in male than in female infants [10]. The high LH and FSH levels during the first 6 months of life in male infants favour the activation of the hypothalamo-pituitary-testicular axis (Fig. 1) [10]. There is a sig-

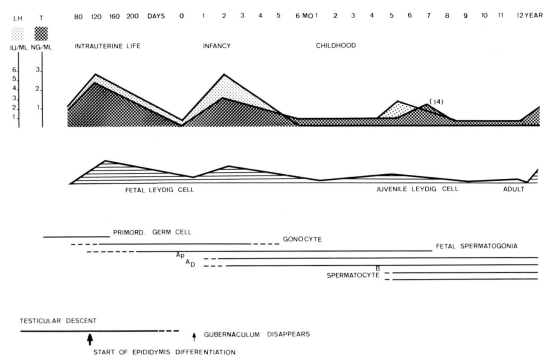

Fig. 1. Development of hypothalamo-pituitary-gonadal axis in correlation to testis development and descent. (*LH*) and testosterone (*T*) values are according to [1, 2, 10, 13]

nificantly higher testosterone rise in premature boys than in full-term boys [11]. This intimates that the active androgen production of the fetal testis in utero advances the maturation of the gonadostat so that maturity is reached earlier in males than in females [11].

From the 7th month onwards and throughout childhood there is a short sluggish interim phase during which the interrelationship between the three components of this regulatory axis are different than in adulthood, namely in the response of the pituitary to GnRH, the gonadal response to HCG and hypothalamic feedback mechanism, and, finally, the plasma sex hormone concentrations [10, 12, 13].

The evident peak of LH secretion, approximately between 4 and 6 years of age, parallels the ultrastructural appearance of the Leydig cells (Fig. 1) [14, 15]. Not only were developed juvenile Leydig cells frequently apparent in this age-group, but also an increase in the number of Sb-Sertoli cells was observed and, for the first time, primary spermatocytes and B spermatogonia are encountered [15]. This indicates that a link exists between the maturation of the

germ, Sertoli, and Leydig cells on the one hand and gonadotropin secretion on the other hand.

In the male the gonad has only an inhibitory effect on the hypothalamo-pituitary-gonadal axis [2]. But the existence of a feedback mechanism in prepuberty is evidently due to:
1. An increase in FSH and compensatory hypertrophy of the descended testis in monorchid and some of the unilateral cryptorchid patients [16].
2. An augmentation in the FSH plasma levels of prepubertal gonadectomized patients [16]

The onset of puberty is genetically determined, but is in the same way related to the maturation of the organism as a whole, particularly of the CNS [17].

The gonadal changes are the result of maturation events occurring at multiple levels of the reproductive hormonal axis which are well summarized by Sverdlov and Heber [17] as follows: At the CNS level, decreasing sensitivity of the gonadostat (hypothalamus), increased stimulatory neurotransmitters production, and pulsatile LH release occur, thus resulting in an increased GnRH release. At the pituitary level, in-

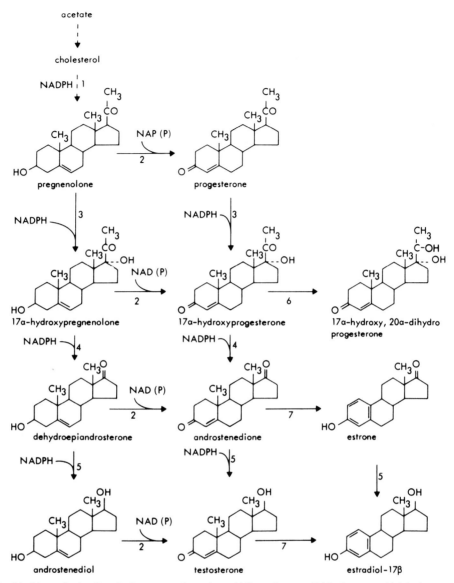

Fig. 2. Pathways involved in biosynthesis of testicular steroids from cholesterol: *1* cholesterol side-chain cleavage complex; *2* 3β-hydroxysteroid dehydrogenase; *3* 17β-hydroxy-lase; *4* steroid C_{1720}-lyase; *5* 17β-hydroxysteroid dehydrogenase; *6* 20α-hydroxysteroid dehydrogenase; *7* aromatizing enzyme complex. (Van der Molen and Rammerts [22])

creased sensitivity of the pituitary to GnRH and an increased LH to FSH ratio in response to GnRH occur. This results in a higher production of gonadotropin, decreased gonad sensitivity to gonadotropin, and changes in androgen biosynthetic pathways. Finally, Sertoli cell maturation also occurs within the testis during this time. As a result of these transformations testosterone production increases and production of mature sperm begins. This raised androgen secretion implies early axillary and pubic hair.

5.3 Role of Leydig Cells

In most mamals the Leydig cells are the main source of testosterone production. Testosterone itself is the main biologically important steroid produced by the testis. In the human fetal testis it has been shown that pregnenolone and dihydroepiandrosterone are present but not progesterone, and it was calculated that in the human fetal testis testosterone formation may occur via pregnenolone, dehydroepiandrosterone, and androstenedione, and not via progesterone [18, 19, 20, 21, 22].

The main precursors for testosterone biosynthesis are fatty acids (Fig. 2). They enter the Leydig cells from the plasma and are degraded to acetyl coenzyme via β oxidation by an enzyme system within the mitochondria [21, 22]. The abundance of smooth endoplasmic reticulum probably reflects the ability of a steroid-secreting cell to produce its own cholesterone rather than taking it up from the plasma [21, 22]. After synthesis the cholesterol is esterified and accumulated in lipoid droplets in the Leydig cell cytoplasm [21]. The cholesterol, destined for testosterone biosynthesis, first enters the mitochondria for cleavage of its side chain. The side-chain cleavage system, involving 20- and 22-hydroxylases and 20, 22-lyase, is presumably located on the mitochondrial inner cristae [21, 22]. Following side-chain cleavage of cholesterol, the resulting 5-pregnenolone must pass through the mitochondrial membrane into the cytoplasm to engage the enzymes necessary for its conversion to testosterone. Three different pathways are known to exist:

1. The progesterone or delta-4 pathway
2. The dehydroepiandrosterone or delta-5 pathway
3. The sulfate pathway

The delta-5 and sulfate pathways appear to be the major routes to the formation of testosterone in the human testis, although low levels of delta-4 intermediates have also been detected [23].

The prepubertal testicular tissue produces metabolites identical to those formed by adult testicular tissue [24, 25].

The steroid metabolic patterns in boys before puberty differ from those found in adults, especially in their dissimilar proportions of newly synthesized 20-alpha-dehydroprogesterone and 17-alpha-hydroxy-progesterone. In testicular tissue below the age of 11 years, 20α-dehydroprogesterone accounts for 40%–80% and 17α-hydroxyprogesterone for only 3%–10% of all metabolites found [25]. In adults and adolescents the proportion of 17α-hydroxyprogesterone rises to 20%–50% [25].

Testosterone may be secreted from the Leydig cells by blood, lymph, or tubular fluid. Blood appears to be quantitatively the most important effluent system because the flow rate is more than 20 times that of lymph and tubular fluids [22]. As there is a good correlation between intracellular and extracellular testicular testosterone, it seems that diffusion is the most important mechanism for testosterone secretion [18, 22, 26].

5.4 Mechanism of Androgen Action

The following summarizes the model for the mechanism of action of androgens in an outstanding contribution by Mainwaring [27]. The testosterone-plasma protein complex, which is stable, enables the testosterone to be transported within the blood. The process by which the testosterone enters all cells is not definitely explained. Particularly within androgen target cells, testosterone will be metabolized extensively into the principal metabolite 5α-dihydrotestosterone (5α-DHT; 17β-hydroxy-5α-androstendian-3-one) [27]. A 17-hydroxy group in the β-plane is mandatory for androgenicity [28] and an oxygen function at the C-3 position is also necessary for its biological activity [27]. The 5α-reductase enzyme necessary for formation of 5α-DHT is basically located in the microsomal fraction [29], but the nuclear fraction [30] and nuclear membrane [31] are also places where it was detected. 5α-DHT is a potent androgen and is specifically bound with a high affinity to a cytoplasmic receptor protein, forming an androgen-receptor protein complex [27].

By stable alterations in the tertiary or quarternary structure, a change in the configuration of the 5α-DHT–receptor protein complex occurs, resulting in an activated complex with an increased propensity for the nuclear acceptor sites. The activated androgen-receptor protein complex is translocated into the nucleus and is retained for a significant but finite period of time at fairly precisely defined sites in chromatin (Fig. 3) [27]. The advent of the androgen-receptor protein complex stimulates many biochemical events that mandatorily require DNA as template, and thereby initiates the spectrum of processes responsible for the manifestation of the androgen response [27]. The hormone-mediated events can be classified as initial, early, and late (Fig. 3) [27]. Initial androgen responses result in enhancement of some ribosomal RNA synthesis, activation of protein phosphokinases, and stimulation of the initiation step of the protein synthesis [27]. The early

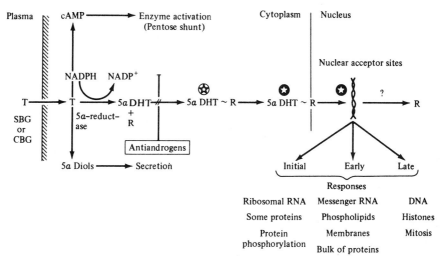

Fig. 3. The mechanism of action of androgens. *T*, testosterone; *SBG*, sex steroid-binding β-globulin; *CBG*, corticosteroid-binding α₂-globulin; *5α-DHT*, 5α-dihydrotestosterone; *5α Diols*, 5α-androstanediols; ✪ and ✪ indicate changes in configuration of receptor complex during activation. (Mainwaring [27])

responses include synthesis of messenger RNA, phospholipids, membranes, and the bulk of proteins, and the late response enhances DNA and histone synthesis and particularly mitosis [27]. The androgen-receptor protein complex finally breaks down or is displaced from the nucleus by an as yet ill-defined mechanism [27]. As a consequence, the critical biochemical processes implicated in the androgen response slow down. The entire system is reversible; interactions between 5α-DHT and the cytoplasmic receptor protein and the subsequent association of the androgen-receptor protein complex with the nuclear acceptor components do not involve covalent bonds [27]. In keeping with this premise, the androgenic steroid remains freely extractable into organic solvents throughout the entire entry and retention process [27].

It was advocated that 5α-DHT specifically controlled cell division, whereas 5α-androstane-3β,17β-diol regulated the secretory process [27]. Macromolecular constituents of all the intercellular organelles are regulated by androgens and the induction of enzymes appears to proceed by an amplification mechanism [27].

Androgens essentially regulate the synthesis of proteins by the provision of more messenger RNA and functional ribosomes. This implies that an enhancement of genetic transcription is the predominant feature of androgenic responses but translational control is also indicated in some studies [27].

Some of the morphological changes in all species promoted by androgens in the target cells are:
1. Mitochondria: depleted and without crista in castrated animals [32, 33]
2. Nucleus, nucleolus: nuclear membrane breaks down and active chromatin disappears after castration; chromatin in perinuclear area without androgen [34]
3. Absorptive organelles (epididymis only): endocytotic vacuoles disappear after castration [35].

Based on the classical model of cell division proposed by Howard and Pelc [36], androgens particularly regulated the duration of the G1 phase. However, in a new concept of cell division in which cells may exist either in an indeterminate A state or a determinate B state [37], androgens would increase the probability of cells entering the B state and hence the process of mitosis [37].

There is evidence that primitive urogenital rudiments are initially insensitive to androgens, later acquiring a hormonal sensitivity that permits the expression of the morphogenic effects of androgenic hormones [38]. The molecular basis of this insensitivity to androgens may be related to the appearance of androgen-receptor proteins in urogenital rudiments [39].

The development of the Wolffian duct and its differentiation requires testosterone. Early fetal castration in both sexes results in female genital duct differentiation [40]. Androgen could influence the development and differentiation of the Wolffian duct, but could not inhibit the Müllerian duct development, indicating the existence of two testicular hormones: androgen and MIS [41]. The findings in anencephalic fetuses with hypoplastic and undescended testes and genitalia, suggest that after the 4th month of gestation HCG is also insufficient to enable gonadal development in the absence of gonadotropin secreted by the fetal pituitary [7]. Also, impairment of the CNS with disturbance of the hypothalamo-pituitary-gonadal axis results in a cryptorchid state (Chap. 4.1).

In the Wolffian ducts no 5α-DHT formation was demonstrable in either sex until the 9.1–11 cm stage of development [42]. This is also the period where no clear epididymis shape is observable. The epididymis is found to begin to acquire its final outline in the 11.5–12.5 cm stage of development. Since in the epididymis the ability to form 5α-DHT was acquired relatively late in the developmental process, testosterone itself is assumed to be the hormone responsible for the initiation of Wolffian duct differentiation [42].

Siiteri and Wilson [42] could not find any significant 5α-DHT formation in the epididymis during embryonal life, whereas a very high rate of 5α-DHT formation was found in the epididymides of adults [43]. Unfortunately, in the crucial phase of the enlargement of the epididymis (after 230 mm C.R.) when testicular descent from the deep inguinal pouch into the scrotum occurs, they examined only an extremely small number of epididymides [42].

In 5α-reductase deficient males, 5α-reductase activity is deficient and the 5α-DHT production in utero is decreased [44]. This results in the development of severe ambiguity of the external genitalia [44]. In the majority of cases cryptorchidism is present [44]. The gross anatomical findings of internal genitalia showed a normal appearance [45, 46, 47, 48]. In puberty, with the elevation of plasma testosterone, the scrotum develops and in the majority of 5α-reductase deficient patients the testes descend [45]. The logical explanation of these cryptorchid states is that due to impaired scrotal development, there is not sufficient space for the testes to descend. But some additional influence of 5α-DHT, particularly on the growth of the epididymis, cannot so far be excluded. Bearing in mind that 5α-DHT influences the mitosis rate in androgen target cells, it may be proposed that 5α-DHT is responsible for enhanced epididymal growth in late fetal life. In particular, the observation that DHT in immature rats may induce testicular descent [49] gives further support to the hypothesis of 5α-DHT influence upon epididymis development.

5.5 Role of Sertoli Cells

As in adults, the Sertoli cell has a supporting and nourishing function. It also serves as a transport regulator and is a part of a blood-testis barrier which probably becomes fully developed only at puberty. The fetal Sertoli cell is particularly well adapted for phagocytosis. The presence of fully developed Sb Sertoli cells seems to have some connection with the appearance of the primary spermatocyte and an intensive development of the Leydig cell in the 4th, 5th, and 6th year. The Sertoli cell is a target cell for FSH, but it is not known to what extent the immature Sertoli cell is involved in hormone production. The Sertoli cell is described as being the source of testicular estrogen production [50]. This occurs by conversion of testosterone into 17β-estradiol under FSH influence [50]. It might have a function in the short loop regulatory system in the testis, and furthermore might be involved in the feedback regulation of gonadotropin secretion [50]. In adult life it plays a local role in the seminiferous tubule by providing suitable conditions for spermatogenesis. In fetal life production of MIS is also ascribed to the Sertoli cells. Several independent research groups believe that "inhibin is also secreted by the Sertoli cells" [51, 52].

5.6 Testing of the Hypothalamo-Pituitary-Gonadal Axis Utilizing GnRH

After its synthesis in 1971 GnRH soon became available for clinical purposes and was immediately used for diagnostic purposes in endocrinology [12]. The first results of various GnRH tests were presented in 1972 and from this time a wide number of publications have been devoted to the diagnostic usefulness of GnRH.

Basal plasma levels of gonadotropin are low in prepubertal children, so they have only limited use as a current index of the gonadotropic function before the onset of puberty [12]. But it is possible to evaluate the gonadotropin pituitary pool and secretion by the intravenous injection of GnRH [12, 13]. Normal children have been studied at different prepubertal and pubertal development stages. In males only the LH response is constant, while there may be a lack of FSH rise to standard stimulation of 0.1 mg/m^2 [13]. Stimulated LH values were higher in male than in female infants, with a maximum in the 1st month of postnatal life [12, 13]. FSH basal and stimulated values were higher in girls than in boys and their releasable stores decrease after 6 months of life [12].

During childhood the LH response to GnRH is similar in boys and girls, but mean FSH response is higher in girls [12, 13]. During puberty in both sexes the LH response increases. FSH response increases similarly in boys, but does not increase with puberty in girls [53]. This has been interpreted to mean that the LH pubertal trend is related only to the maturation of the negative hypothalamic feedback or gonadostat, while the FSH trend is probably related also to the different feedback effects of male and female gonadal steroids, although no increase in FSH in pubertal boys was reported [13, 53, 54]. These discrepancies may result in part from different amounts of GnRH administered. Grumbach and co-workers have demonstrated that augmenting doses of GnRH from 1 to 200 µg/m^2 body weight increases the response of both gonadotropins in boys [55]. In general today, the 100 µg i.v. dose for studies of hypothalamo-pituitary-gonadal axis in boys is recommended [56]. With this dose, maximal evaluation of releasable gonadotropin stores in prepubertal patients occurs. Furthermore, the use of a constant infusion of GnRH (100 µg in a 3 h infusion) has been advocated [57]. Utilizing of GnRH has had no side effect and no such adverse effect has been reported in any relevant literature.

5.7 Development of the Hypothalamo-Pituitary-Gonadal Axis in Cryptorchid Boys

The involvement of testosterone in the etiology of cryptorchidism is already evident between 2 and 6 months after birth. At this stage there is a diminished or nonexistent increase in testosterone plasma levels in true cryptorchid boys (Fig. 4) [58]. This was observed in a cross-sectional study [58]. A longitudinal study of testosterone secretion in the first year has also been published. The concentration of the three components of the retinol circulating complex demonstrates in healthy male infants, but not in females, a transient elevation cumulating at 5–6 months after birth [59]. This trimolecular peak is significantly less elevated in bilateral cryptorchid babies [59]. The rise of retinol-related parameters seems directly induced by the testosterone hypersecretion previously described in male infants at 2–3 months of age [59]. Thus these latter observations parallel the already-observed atrophic appearance of Leydig cells in cryptorchid infants [60]. It is generally accepted that the basal plasma testosterone, which is low in the prepubertal period, is within the normal range in boys with undescended testes (for review see 24). However, the involvement of testosterone secretion in the pathogenesis of cryptorchidism becomes clearly apparent if the Leydig cells are stimulated with HCG. A proper dose, number of injections, and rhythm is thus important. For example, if high doses of HCG are used ($9 \times 1,500$ IU instead of $3 \times 1,500$ IU), a more sustained stimulation could cancel out the difference between cryptorchids and controls [61]. In the past 10 years numerous reports on impaired testosterone rise after HCG stimulation in uni- or bilateral cryptorchids have been made (for review see 24). One of the significant findings was that there is no correlation between the incidence of abnormal response to HCG and an occurrence of uni- or bilateral cryptorchidism. Derived from her data, Forest [24] suggests that Leydig cell damage may affect both testes in a case of unilateral cryptorchidism, rather than being a direct consequence of the malposition of the undescended testis. In contrast to the impaired secretion, an abnormal biosynthesis of testosterone was not encountered in crypt-

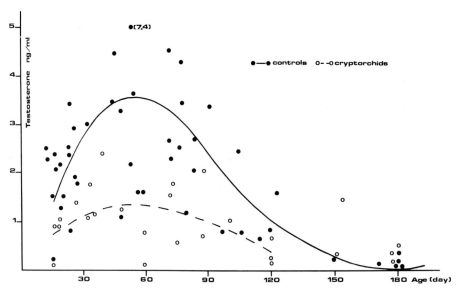

Fig. 4. Plasma testosterone in cryptorchid and normal boys. (Gendrel et al. [13])

orchid boys [24, 25]. Although the Leydig and Sertoli cell functions of undescended testes are similar to those in normally descended testes, the mean concentration of cAMP in descended testes was significantly lower (in basal condition) than in undescended testes, further indicating an impaired stimulation of Leydig cells in cryptorchid boys [62].

Since response to HCG becomes normal at the mid-puberty stage, this indicates a delay in the maturation of Leydig cells to respond to LH and/or HCG stimulation [61]. The delayed response was noted not only for testosterone, but also for estrogens [61].

In contrast to these findings, several reports show that this impairment in testosterone secretion remains in a percentage of cryptorchid males for life [63]. Engberg found a significantly decreased amount of androgens in the urine of bilateral cryptorchid adults [63]. Identical observations were made by Raboch and Starka [64]. The fact that only about $^1/_{16}$ of normal testicular tissue is necessary for the development of normal secondary sex characteristics [65] makes it clear why cryptorchid men may have such characteristics even with diminished androgen secretion. The undescended testis can occur in panhypopituitarism, hypogonadotrophic hypogonadism, and Kallman's syndrome. Clinical experience is that the boy with gonadotropin deficiency is usually character-

ized by sexual infantilism, which may manifest as micropenis, an underdeveloped scrotum, and/or cryptorchidism.

In cryptorchid boys LH basal levels and response to GnRH are significantly lower from infancy to early puberty than in boys with normally descended testes [66]. In recent years this observation has been confirmed several times [67–70, 72] although a negative report does exist [71]. Most of the reports, however, describe that in at least some cryptorchid boys or adults there is a partial LH deficiency. When GnRH infusions were performed, a deficiency of the hypothalamo-pituitary-gonadal axis was shown to exist in most cryptorchid boys [70]. Sixty-nine boys [bone age 2–10 years, puberty rating I (Tanner)] with unilateral or bilateral cryptorchidism, admitted for orchidopexy, underwent a GnRH test in our clinic. The mean basal LH was 4.3 ± 2.2 mIU/ml and the mean peak response to LH was 6.6 mIU/ml. These results did not differ from data for normal boys of the same age. The mean basal FSH value in cryptorchid boys studied was 1.3 ± 0.7 mIU/ml with a mean peak value of 4.43 mIU/ml. This also accords with normal FSH values.

A correlation between histological and endocrinological values in cryptorchid boys underlines the impairment of their reproductive axis. When group A of unilateral cryptorchid prepubertal boys (S/T = 0) was compared to group B

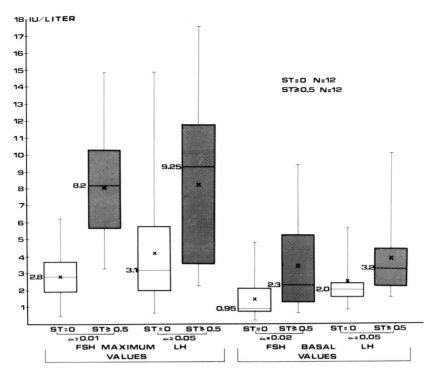

Fig. 5. LH and FSH basal and peak plasma values in two groups of unilateral cryptorchid boys. The *lines* in the bars represent mean values, *x* denotes arithmetical mean, and *bars* denote interquartile range

(S/T > 0.5), there was a significant difference in both LH and FSH values. At the same time, group B also had a higher number of germ cells in the contralateral descended gonad (Fig. 12, Chap. 4).

The low LH and FSH basal and stimulation plasma values, despite the presence of more severely damaged testes, point to hypogonadotropic hypogonadism being more expressed in group A although they had the same age and position of the gonads as group B. Although gonadal damage was universal in cryptorchid boys, only 22% of these boys had a rise in basal gonadotropins, particularly FSH (Table 1) (Fig. 5). An impaired increase in FSH is to be interpreted as a result of hypothalamo-pituitary dysfunction.

Since almost all cryptorchid boys have a normal puberty, it is clear that the underlaying gonadotropin deficit must be incomplete. According to Canlorbe et al. it should disappear after puberty [61].

Until puberty the cytoplasmic appearance of the Sertoli cells, particularly in the Sf and Sb stages, shows that they all have conditions favourable to hormone production (lamellar bodies, smooth and rough endoplasmic reticulum). The extensive histometric studies of the Sertoli cells and correlation to gonadotropins performed in our laboratory have failed to link gonadotropins with the Sertoli cells [73]. The mean number of Sertoli cells in 25 cryptorchid patients (P_1 stage of puberty) was 38.93 ± 7.8 tubule. The count of degenerating

Table 1. Basal values for LH and FSH from eight controls and 53 unilateral cryptorchid boys (mean ± SD)

	S/T control ≥ 2	S/T = 0	S/T > 0 < 0.5	S/T ≥ 0.5
LH (mIU/ml)	4.3 ± 2.2	2.5 ± 2.2	3.9 ± 1.9	4.0 ± 2.7
FSH (mIU/ml	1.3 ± 0.7	1.5 ± 1.3	1.36 ± 0.89	3.4 ± 2.9
No. of patients and % of distribution		12 (22%)	29 (56%)	12 (22%)

Sertoli cells was 26.5% (10.35 ± 7.26) of all the cells in each seminiferous tubule. There was no correlation between the number of degenerating Sertoli cells and gonadotropins, either in basal or stimulated plasma values. The histometric results thus obtained have also confirmed the already-promulgated lack of difference in the number of degenerated Sertoli cells in normal and cryptorchid boys [15].

References

1. Winter AJ, Eskay RL, Porter JC (1974) Concentration and distribution of TRH and LRH in the fetal brain. J Clin Endocrinol Metab 39:960–963
2. Kaplan LS, Grumbach MM (1976) The ontogenesis of human foetal hormones. II. Luteinizing hormone (LH) and follicle stimulating hormone (FSH). Acta Endocrinol 81:808–829
3. Furukashi N, Suzuki M, Fukaya T, Kono H, Tachibana J, Shinkawa O (1980) Effects of synthetic LH-RH and TRH on pituitary function in anencephalic infants. Gynecol Obstet Invest 11:231–236
4. Chin KY (1938) The endocrine glands of anencephalic foetuses. Chin Med J [Suppl 2] 63–90
5. Zondek LH, Zondek T (1965) Observations on the testis in anencephaly with special references to the Leydig cells. Biol Neonat 8:329–347
6. Bearn JG (1968) Anencephaly and the development of the male genital tract. Acta Pediatr Acad Sci (Hung) 9:159–180
7. Baker GT, Scrimgeour BJ (1980) Development of the gonad in normal and anencephalic human fetuses. J Reprod Fertil 60:193–199
8. Faiman Ch, Winter SDJ, Reyes IF (1981) Endocrinology of the fetal testis. In: Burger H, Kretser D de (eds), The testis. Raven Press, New York
9. Gulyas BJ, Tullner WW, Hodgen GD (1977) Fetal or maternal hypophysectomy in rhesus monkeys (Macaca mulatta): Effects on the development of the testes and other endocrine organs. Biol Reprod 17:650–660
10. Forest GM, Saez MJ, Bertrand J (1973) Assessment of gonadal function in children. Pediatrician 2:102–128
11. Tapainen J, Koivisto M, Vihko R, Huhtaniemi I (1981) Enhanced activity of the pituitary-gonadal axis in premature human infants. J Clin Endocrinol Metab 52:235–238
12. Job JC, Chaussain JL, Garnier PE (1977) The use of luteinizing hormone-releasing hormone in pediatric patients. Hormone Res 8:171–187
13. Job JC, Pierson M (1981) Endocrinologie pédiatrique et croissance. Flammarion médecine-sciences, Paris
14. Waaler PE: Morphometric studies in undescended testes. In: Job Cl (ed), Cryptorchidism. Pediatric Adolescent Endocrinology. Karger, Basel
15. Hadžiselimović F (1977) Cryptorchidism. Springer, Heidelberg Berlin New York
16. Tatò L, Masè R, Pinelli L, Pizzo P, Gaburro D (1979) Monorchism. In: Job JC (ed) Cryptorchidism, diagnosis and treatment. Karger, Basel, pp 148–153
17. Swerdloff SR, Heber D (1981) Endocrine control of testicular function from birth to puberty. In: Burger H, Kretser D de (eds) The testis. Raven Press, New York
18. Eik-Nes KB (1970) The androgens of the testis. Marcel Dekker, New York
19. Wilson JD (1975) Metabolism of testicular androgens. In: Greep OR, Astwook BE (eds) Handbook of Physiology, sect 7/V. American Physiological Society, Washington D.C.
20. Ewing L, Brown BL (1977) Testicular steroidogenesis. In: Johnson DA, Gomes RW (eds) The testis, vol IV. Academic Press, New York
21. Tsang BK, Kinson AG (1980) Biogenesis of androgens and estrogens by the normal testis. In: Hafez ESE (ed) Descended and cryptorchid testis. Martinus Nijhoff, The Hague, Boston London
22. Molen JH van der, Rammerts GFF (1981) Testicular steroidogenesis. In: Burger H, Kretser D de (eds) The testis. Raven Press, New York
23. Yanaihava T, Troën P (1972) Studies of the human testis. I. Biosynthetic pathways for androgen formation in human testicular tissue in vitro. J Clin Endocrinol Metab 34:783–792
24. Forest GM (1971) Pattern of the response to HCG stimulation in prepubertal cryptorchid boys. In: Job Cl (ed) Cryptorchidism. Pediatric Adolescent Endocrinology. Karger, Basel
25. Berg AA, Lackgren G, Lundkrist K (1979) Androgen biosynthesis in cryptorchid and non-cryptorchid human testicular tissue. In: Bierich RJ, Giarola A (eds) Cryptorchidism. Academic Press, London New York Toronto Sidney San Francisco
26. Parvinen M, Hurme P, Niemi M (1970) Penetration of exogenous testosterone, pregnenolone, progesterone and cholesterol into the seminiferous tubulus of the rat. Endocrinology 87:1082–1084
27. Mainwaring WIP (1977) The mechanism of action of androgens. Springer, New York Heidelberg Berlin
28. Liao S, Liang T, Fang S, Casteñeda E, Shao TC (1973) Steroid structure and androgenic activity. Specifities involved in the receptor binding and nuclear retention of various androgens. J Biol Chem 248:6154–6162
29. Chamberlain J, Jagovinec C, Ofner P (1966) Catabolism of [4-^{14}C] testosterone by subcellular fractions of human prostate. Biochem J 99:610–616
30. Bruchovsky N, Wilson JD (1968) The conversion of testosterone to 5α-androstol-17-β-a-3-one by rat prostate in vivo and in vitro. J Biol Chem 243:2012–2021
31. Moore RJ, Wilson JD (1972) Localization of the reduced nicotinamide adenine dinucleotide phosphate: Δ^4-3-ketosteroid 5α-oxidoreductase in the nuclear membrane of rat ventral prostate. J Biol Chem 247:958–967
32. Allison VF (1964) Ultrastructural changes in the seminal vesicle epithelium of the rat following castration and androgen stimulation. Anat Rec 148:254
33. Orlandini G (1964) Effects of castration on mitochondria structure in accessory glands of the mouse. Arch Ital Anat Embriolog 71:149
34. Brandes D (1974) Fine structure and cytochemistry of male accessory sex organs. In: Brandes D (ed) Male accessory sex organs. Academic Press, New York
35. Nicander L (1965) An electron microscopic study of absorbing cells in the posterior caput epididymidis of rabbits. Z Zellforsch 66:829–847
36. Howard A, Pelc SR (1951) Nuclear incorporation of

p^{32} as demonstrated by autoradiography. Exp Cell Res 2:178–187

37. Smith JA, Martin L (1973) Do cell cycle? Proc Natl Acad Sci USA 70:1263

38. Ohno S (1977) Testosterone and cellular response. In: Blandau RJ, Bergsma D (eds) Morphogenesis and malformation of the genital system. Liss, New York

39. Cunia RG, Lung B (1979) Development of male accessory gland. In: Hafez ESE (ed) Accessory glands of the male reproductive tract. Spring-Mills, E., Ann Arbor Science

40. Jost A (1946) Sur la différenciation sexuelle de l'embryon de lapin. Expériences de paraboise. CR Soc Biol 140:463–464

41. Donahue RP, Ito Y, Marfatia S, Hendren HW (1976) The production of Müllerian Inhibiting Substance by the fetal, neonatal and adult rat. Biol Reprod 15:329–334

42. Siiteri KP, Wilson DJ (1974) Testosterone formation and metabolism during male sexual differentiation in the human embryo. J Clin Endocrinol Metab 38:113–122

43. Gloyna RE, Wilson DJ (1969) A comparative study of the conversion of testosterone to 17β-hydroxy-5α-androstan-3-one (Dihydrotestosterone) by prostate and epididymis. J Clin Endocrinol Metab 29:970–977

44. Imperato-McGinley J, Guerrero L, Gautier T, Peterson RE (1974) Steroid 5α-reductase deficiency in man: An inherited form of male pseudohermaphroditism. Science 186:1213–1215

45. Peterson ER, Imperato-McGinley J, Gautier T, Sturla E (1977) Male Pseudohermaphroditism due to steroid 5α-reductase deficiency. Am J Med 62:170–191

46. Imperato-McGinley J, Peterson ER, Gautier T, Sturla E (1979) Androgens and the evolution of male-gender identity among male pseudohermaphrodites with 5α-reductase deficiency. N Engl J Med 300:1233–1237

47. Walsh CP, Madden DJ, Harrod JM, Goldstein LJ, MacDonald CP, Wilson DJ (1974) Familial incomplete male pseudohermaphroditism, Type 2. N Engl J Med 290:944–949

48. Fisher KL, Kogut DM, Moore JR, Dobelsman U, Weitzman JJ, Isaacs HJr, Griffin EJ, Wilson DJ (1978) Clinical, endocrinological, and enzymatic characterization of two patients with 5α-reductase deficiency: Evidence that a single enzyme is responsible for the 5α-reduction of cortisol and testosterone. J Clin Endocrinol Metab 47:653–664

49. Raifer J, Walsh PC (1977) Testicular descent. In: Blandau RJ, Bergsma D (eds) Birth Defects. Original Article Series, Vol 13, No 2. Morphogenesis and Malformation of the Genital System. Liss, New York

50. Dorrington JH, Fritz B, Armstrong DT (1976) Testicular estrogens; Synthesis by isolated Sertoli cells and regulation by follicles-stimulating hormone. In: Spielman CH, Lobl TJ, Kirton RT (eds) Regulatory mechanisms of male reproductive physiology. Excerpta Medica American Elsevier, Amsterdam Oxford New York

51. Franchimont P, Chori S, Hagelstein MT, Puraiswami S (1975) Existence of a follicle-stimulating hormone inhibiting factor, "inhibin" in bull seminal plasma. Nature (Lond) 257:402–404

52. Setschell PB, Davis VR, Main JS (1977) Inhibin. In: Johnson DA, Gomes RW (eds) The testis, IV. Academic Press, New York San Francisco London

53. Suwa S, Maesaka H, Matsui I (1974) Serum LH and FSH responses to synthetic LH-RH in normal infants, children, and patients with Turner's syndrome. Pediatrics 54:470–475

54. Roth JC, Kelch RP, Kaplan SL, Grumbach MM (1972) FSH and LH response to luteinizing hormone-releasing factor in prepubertal and pubertal children, adult males and patients with hypogonadotropic and hypergonadotropic hypogonadism. J Clin Endocrinol Metab 35:926–930

55. Grumbach MM, Roth JC, Kaplan SL, Kelch RP (1974) Hypothalamic pituitary regulation of puberty in man. Evidence and concepts derived from clinical research. In: Grumbach MM, Grave DG, Mayer EF (eds) The control of the onset of puberty. Wiley, New York

56. Wollesen F, Swerdloff RS, Odell WD (1976) LH and FSH responses to luteinizing-releasing hormone in normal adult human males. Metabolism 25:845–863

57. Reiter EO, Root AW, Duckett GE (1976) The response of pituitary gonadotropes to a constant infusion of LHRH in normal prepubertal and pubertal children and in children with abnormalities of sexual development. J Clin Endocrinol Metab 43:400

58. Gendrel D, Job JCl, Roger M (1978) Reduced postnatal rise of testosterone in plasma of cryptorchid infants. Acta Endocrinol 89:372–378

59. Ingenbleck Y, Hoven FM van den, Deruelle M (1981) Differences in the retinol circulating complex between healthy male and female infants. Clinica Chimica Acta 114:219–224

60. Hadžiselimović F, Herzog B, Seguchi H (1975) Surgical correction of cryptorchidism at 2 years. Electron microscopic and morphometric investigations. J Pediat Surg 10:19–28

61. Canlorbe P, Toublanc JE, Roger M, Job JCl (1974) Etude de la fonction endocrine dans 125 cas de cryptorchidies. Ann Med Interne 125:365

62. Lloyd III JW, Stecker JF, Rakestraw MG (1978) In vitro stimulation of adenosine 3′,5′-monophosphate in unilateral undescended testes of humans by follicle and luteinizing hormone. J Clin Endocrinol Metab 46:158–162

63. Engberg H (1949) Investigations of the endocrine function of the testicle in cryptorchidism. Proc R Soc Med 42:652–655

64. Raboch J, Starka L (1972) Plasmatic testosterone in bilateral cryptorchids in adult age. Andrologie 4:107–112

65. Lipschütz A, Ottow B (1920) Sur les conséquences de la castration partielle. CR Soc Biol (Paris) 83:1340

66. Job C, Garnier PhE, Chaussain JL, Toublanc JE, Canlorbe P (1974) Effect of synthetic luteinizing hormone-releasing hormone on the release of gonadotropins in hypophyso-gonadal disorders of children and adolescents. IV. Undescended testes. J Pediatr 84:371–374

67. Jacobelli A, Agosto A, Vecci E, Simeoni A, Ferantelli M (1979) Studies on the pituitary-testicular axis in boys with cryptorchidism. In: Bierich JR, Giarolla A (eds) Cryptorchidism. Academic Press, London

68. Mazzi C, Riva LP, Morandi G, Mainini E, Scarsi G, Salaroli A (1979) A study of cryptorchid subjects. I. Evaluation of the hypophyseal-testicular axis in the prepubertal period. In: Bierich JR, Giarolla A (eds) Cryptorchidism. Eds.: Academic Press, London

69. Tatò L, Masé R, Rossignoli R, Pinelli L, Gaburro D (1979) Some semiological aspects of cryptorchidism in prepubertal boys. Testicular volume and gonadotropin responses to LH-RH. In: Bierich JR, Giarolla A (eds) Cryptorchidism. Academic Press, London

70. Vanelli N, Bernasconi R, Vipdis R, Giovannelli G (1981) Gonadotropine response to 3 hours LHRH infusion in cryptorchid and normal children. Pediatr Res 15:88

71. Cacciari E, Cicognani A, Pirazzoli P, Zappola F, Tassoni P, Bernardi F, Salardi S (1976) Hypophysogon-adal function in the cryptorchid children. Difference between unilateral and bilateral cryptorchidism. Acta Endocrinol [Copenh] 83:182–189

72. Happ J (1981) Therapie mit Gonadotropin-Releasing-Hormon. Urban & Schwarzenberg, München Wien Baltimore

73. Rehorek R (1982) Die Beziehung der Sertoli-Zelle zu der hypothalamo-hypophyso-gonadalen Achse bei kryptorchen präpubertalen Knaben. Inaugural-Dissertation der Medizinischen Universität Basel

6 Fertility in Cryptorchidism

S.J. Kogan

"....prevailing methods of treatment of cryptorchidism are unsatisfactory and ... boys with ... cryptorchidism ... should be spared the hazard and inconvenience of orchidopexy"
(Charny)

6.1 Introduction

It is common knowledge that the testis that remains cryptorchid through puberty will be sterile later in life. However, a number of patients who are treated prepubertally, even with unilateral cryptorchidism, will also be infertile in adulthood. At a conservative estimate, some 25% of unilateral and 50% of bilateral cryptorchids will be infertile in spite of successful prepubertal orchidopexy.

In 1960, Charny [1] made the following statement:

"Testicular biopsy in a large number of testes brought into the scrotum by a variety of techniques failed to reveal a single instance of normal spermatogenesis .... prevailing methods of treatment of cryptorchidism are not satisfactory and the operative techniques, as practised by most surgeons, yield better cosmetic than functional results. If the surgical technique cannot be improved sufficiently, boys with asymptomatic cryptorchidism without clinically recognized hernia should be spared the hazard and inconvenience of orchidopexy".

Charny's pessimistic view stands as a challenge to all those who treat cryptorchidism to improve upon the results of treatment. If we are to do so, it is important to understand the reason for the impaired fertility that is seen. Most important, it is necessary to understand that patients with cryptorchidism do not constitute one uniform group with a single underlying cause of the infertility, but rather are a heterogeneous group with diverse underlying causes.

6.2 Factors Influencing the Interpretation of Infertility Data in Cryptorchid Patients

Numerous series have been published analyzing the incidence of infertility in medically and surgically treated adults with previously treated cryptorchidism; however, evaluation of the results cited in these series is difficult. Considerable variation is evident. Some of the factors causing difficulty with direct comparison are:

1. Source of patients, i.e., random, infertility clinic, etc.
2. Exclusion of some patients from results
3. Age at treatment
4. HCG ± surgery
5. Location of testis
6. Inclusion of retractile testes
7. Injury at surgery
8. Technique of sperm analysis
9. Definition of Infertility

Certain points bear re-emphasis.

6.2.1 Patient Source

Considerable heterogeneity exists in the patient composition of different series. In some series, patient source is not mentioned. In others, analysis of patients from infertility clinics are included in results, obviously a negative influence. Screening for Kleinfelter's syndrome, which occurs with a reported incidence of 1:88 in the pediatric cryptorchid population, a five-fold increase over the normal incidence [2], is usually not done or not specified.

6.2.2 Age at Treatment

Age at treatment has been shown to be of importance, since progressive histologic deterioration occurs with increasing age, yet in many instances it is not specified in retrospective analyses. Some series collate all patients treated at different ages into one general grouping. In at least two series, early treatment correlated directly with subsequent fertility [3, 4].

6.2.3 Medical VS Surgical Treatment

In most series of patients treated with HCG, later analysis shows fertility to be greater than in surgically treated patients. Method of treatment therefore influences results, and inclusion of varying numbers of medically treated patients or patients failing medical treatment affects analysis of fertility results achieved.

6.2.4 Location of Testis

In more recent series analyzing fertility in cryptorchidism, an effort has been made to exclude patients having retractile testes. This distinction is important, since the latter have been shown to have normal testicular development and subsequent fertility [5]. Yet in spite of these attempts, this distinction may sometimes not be achievable, as shown by analysis of a recent collaborative series regarding treatment of undescended testes where retractile testes were included in spite of careful attempts by experienced observers to exclude them [6].

Few series cite the location of the undescended testis prior to treatment and then correlate the results of treatment with subsequent fertility. However, it is known that the high or intra-ababdominal testis is more difficult to bring into the scrotum, by either medical or surgical means, and that results in terms of fertility are worse in this group. Series having fewer or greater numbers of patients having high testes included cannot be meaningfully compared.

6.2.5 Injury from Surgery

Many series do not state whether evaluation of testis size or location following surgery, two obvious measures of surgical success, have been done. Published reports indicate up to 40% atrophy in some series, making assessment of subsequent fertility in these patients inaccurate [7].

At best, a 2% incidence of atrophy following primary orchidopexy and a 1% incidence of vas injury in similar patients have been described [8, 9]. Surgical technique would seem to influence results to a greater extent in some series, especially in those including more patients with difficult orchidopexies.

Though a palpably good result regarding testis size and location correlates with fertility, some testes meeting this criteria will ultimately be sterile. A poor anatomic result is invariably associated with infertility.

6.2.6 Method of Sperm Analysis

A lack of uniformity of methodology in performing semen analysis is evident in reviewing extant fertility data in cryptorchid patients. Most series do not comment on whether one or more specimens have been obtained, nor do they mention the period of abstinence prior to collection. The latter, in particular, is important [10] and has been shown to result in significant alterations in individual counts in cryptorchid patients [11].

6.2.7 Definition of Infertility

Interpretation of infertility data in published series of cryptorchid patients requires a common definition of infertility. In many series, the accepted arbitrary definition of 20 million sperm/cc by semen analysis has been used [12]; in others, a lower count has been accepted. Neither value may be a true indication of infertility, as lower counts are compatible with fertilization [10].

Documentation of motility and morphology becomes important at lower counts, but are seldom mentioned. Rather than referring to infertility, reference to mean sperm density in these cryptorchid patients appears to be a more accurate way to describe the impairment.

In some series, fertility has been measured by paternity. This measurement is fraught with obvious problems and appears in general to overestimate the true incidence of fertility [13].

Taking these factors into account explains some of the variation in fertility results seen between published series. However, it is clear that in both unilateral and bilateral cryptorchidism a defect exists, adversely affecting subsequent fertility.

6.3 Analysis of Extant Fertility Data

Analysis of more recent series of cryptorchid patients published during the last 10 years has allowed for more accurate assessment of the true incidence of impaired fertility. A reanalysis of the recorded data from 11 recent series of unbilateral cryptorchids and nine series of bilateral cryptorchids is shown in Tables 1 and 2. In these tables only more recent series have been analyzed, since evaluation of cryptorchid patients in these series has been performed with better understanding and more careful attention, and has tended to be much more precise. The mean incidence of fertility in bilateral cryptorchid patients is 28% (range 8%–48%); in unilateral cryptorchids it is 51.5% (range 25%–81%). This sharply contrasts with the often-quoted figure of 10% fertility amongst couples, to which the male partner may be a primary or contributing cause half of the time (*W.H.O. Statistics,* 1969) [14].

6.4 Special Considerations Regarding Fertility in Cryptorchidism

Three special considerations are important in the understanding of the pathogenesis of infertility in cryptorchidism: the association of successful HCG-induced descent and subsequent fertility; the relation of compensatory testicular hypertrophy and fertility; and the evidence that a unilateral pathologic testis may induce functional and histologic changes in the normal testis. Investigations in the latter field, in particular, have given startling new insights into the infertility process.

6.5 Correlation of HCG-Induced Descent and Subsequent Fertility

In non-North American centers where many cryptorchid boys have historically been treated first with HCG rather than surgery, long experience and follow-up has allowed for correlation of testicular descent using HCG and subsequent fertility. A direct correlation was shown between successful descent utilizing HCG and fertility in an adult follow-up of 66 men [15]. Histologic abnormalities shown in the biopsies

Table 1. Fertility (20 million sperm/cc) in unilateral cryptorchidism

Authors	Year	n	F/I	Fertile (%)
Madersbacher et al. [40]	1972	36	9/25	25
Schreiber et al. [41]	1976	66	32/34	48
Werder et al. [42]	1976	23	13/10	57
Lipschultz [43]	1976	29	21/8	72
Richter et al. [28]	1976	28	15/13	53.5
Retief et al. [44]	1977	76	52/24	68
Scheiber et al. [35]	1979	46	13/33	39
Dickerman[a] et al. [18]	1979	47	18/29	38
Knorr[a] et al. [46]	1979	72	33/39	46
Wojciechowski et al. [45]	1979	106	55/46	49.5
Zamudio-Albescu[a] [26]	1979	32	18/29	38
		561	281/280	Range 25–81% Mean 51.5%

[a] Fertility defined as 12 million sperm/cc
(F/I) F = fertile, I = infertile males

Table 2. Fertility (20 million sperm/cc) in bilateral cryptorchidism

Authors	Year	n	F/I	Fertile (%)
Czaplicki et al. [47]	1974	36	20/16	55
Bramble et al. [48]	1974	21	10/11	48
Richter et al. [28]	1976	50	19/31	38
Werder et al. [42]	1976	14	3/11	21
Retief et al. [44]	1977	29	10/19	34
Dickerman et al. [18]	1979	21	2/19	9.5
Knorr[a] et al. [46]	1979	49	14/49	28.5
Wojciechowsky et al. [45]	1979	48	7/41	14.5
Scheiber et al. [35]	1981	36	3/33	8
		281	72/209	Range 8–48% Mean 28.5%

[a] Fertility defined as 12 million sperm/cc
F = fertile, I = infertile males (F/I)

Table 3. Fertility in adults treated only with HCG and in those treated with HCG and subsequent surgery. Numbers in parentheses are percentages. (Bierich [18])

	Fertile	Subfertile	Infertile	
Fertility after successful HCG treatment
Unilateral	43	23 (53)	14 (33)	6 (14)
Bilateral	35	13 (37)	11 (31)	11 (31)
Total	78	36 (46)	25 (32)	17 (22)
Fertility after unsuccessful HCG treatment and subsequent operation
Unilateral	28	9 (32)	12 (43)	7 (25)
Bilateral	15	2 (13)	3 (20)	10 (67)
Total	43	11 (25)	15 (35)	17 (40)

of the cryptorchid testes undergoing orchidopexy immediately following unsuccessful HCG treatment correlated with subsequent infertility [16]. In a larger series reporting a follow-up spermatologic investigation of 121 men treated for undescended testes before puberty, the fertility in those testes not descending with HCG was about half as much as in the HCG-responsive group (Table 3). Unilateral and bilateral cryptorchid individuals showed a similar reduction [17, 18]. Though small numbers of retractile testes, which are uniformly responsive to HCG and have good histopathology, could conceivably have been included in these series, inclusion of these few patients could hardly result in the halving of the fertility rate observed. Rather, it appears that the unsuccessful response to HCG can select out the qualitatively inferior testes with a poorer prognosis. These observations also explain the lessened fertility rate reported in surgically treated patients, as they often represent HCG treatment failures.

6.6 Fertility in Cryptorchid Patients with Compensatory Testicular Hypertrophy

Compensatory hypertrophy of a descended testis (CTH) may occur when the other testis is absent, damaged, or undescended (Fig. 1). It has been estimated to occur in 6%–12% of unilaterally cryptorchid boys [19, 20].

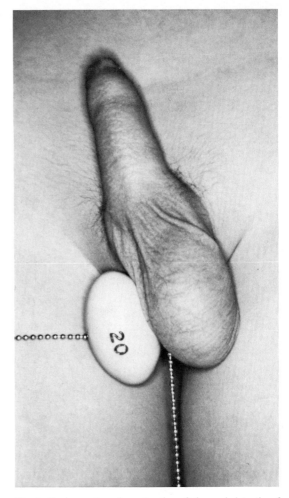

Fig. 1. Compensatory hypertrophy of descended testis of unilaterally cryptorchid boy, age 12 years. Testis of 20 ml, represents 99th percentile. At age 13 2/12ths years, testis had grown to 50 ml

Development of CTH has been considered as a favorable sign, that the descended testis could normally respond to the excess gonadotropin secretion resulting from loss of inhibition by the contralateral damaged (or absent) testis. This would seem physiologic and analogous to situations in which other paired organs, i.e., kidneys, undergo compensatory hypertrophy to compensate for loss of or damage to the other. Experimentally produced CTH and human CTH are generally associated with hypersecretion of FSH [20, 21] (Fig. 2). A recent endocrinologic evaluation of prepubertal unilateral cryptorchid boys with and without CTH revealed that boys with CTH demonstrated a higher than normal LH secretion after LHRH

Fig. 2. FSH levels in rats with compensatory testicular hypertrophy experimentally produced by hemicastration. Weight of testis in controls = 612 mg, weight of remaining testis in hemiorchiectomized rats with CTH = 716 mg; $P < 0.005$. (Kogan SJ, Smey P, Levitt SB, unpublished data, 1979)

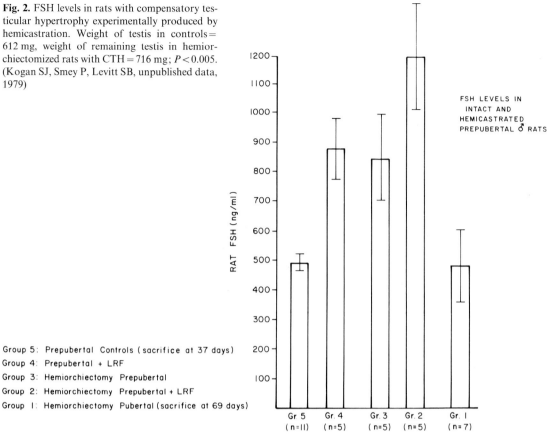

Group 5: Prepubertal Controls (sacrifice at 37 days)
Group 4: Prepubertal + LRF
Group 3: Hemiorchiectomy Prepubertal
Group 2: Hemiorchiectomy Prepubertal + LRF
Group 1: Hemiorchiectomy Pubertal (sacrifice at 69 days)

stimulation, and a higher testosterone secretion after HCG; whereas in the cryptorchid boys without CTH, both responses were subnormal. These responses suggest that different mechanisms are operative in these two groups of cryptorchids [19].

Even if CTH is a phenomenon occurring in normal testes, the ultimate fertility capacity may be diminished in adulthood. A recent follow-up of seven adults showing evidence of CTH who had previously corrected unilateral cryptorchidism demonstrated that in spite of development of CTH their fertility was impaired. Of the seven, five had less than 20 million sperm/cc, and two had complete azospermia [20]. It may be that the occurrence of CTH represents an abnormal response, i.e., the descended testis should normally be able to inhibit FSH hypersecretion, which is associated with the development of CTH. Lack of inhibition would be the finding in an abnormal descended testis, with CTH occurring as a

result. Corroborating evidence confirming which of these theories is correct will require adult follow-up of additional patients showing evidence of CTH.

6.7 Evidence for a Contralateral Lesion in the Descended Testis

The impaired fertility seen in unilateral cryptorchids raises the suspicion of a bilateral lesion being present, affecting the descended testis as well. This lesion might result from a primary abnormality similar to that seen in the undescended testis, a secondary response to the presence of the undescended testis, or both. A growing body of evidence now exists that both congenital and acquired abnormalities may be associated with development of abnormalities in the descended "normal" testis.

A diminished number of germ cells in the descended testes of unilaterally cryptorchid

boys has been described by several investigators, in up to two-thirds of the cases in one
series [22]. The explanation of why one testis
descends and the other does not remains
unclear, though generally the germ cell counts
in the descended testis (though diminished) are
higher than those observed in the undescended
one [23]. In up to 40% of patients with unilateral cryptorchidism, the total germ cell counts
from biopsies of both testes do not exceed the
numbers found in bilaterally cryptorchid cases,
indicating a deficiency in both testes [24].

Experimentally, production of unilateral orchitis [25, 26], unilateral testicular torsion [27],
and unilateral cryptorchidism [28, 29, 30] have
been reported to cause histologic abnormalities
in the contralateral testis. In one elegant study
of the effects of unilateral testicular torsion in
which fertility was directly evaluated in a rat
model by subsequent mating tests, 24 h torsion
resulted in reduction of fertility to zero. When
the twisted testis was resected after 24 h, subsequent fertility was restored to 86% of normal
[31].

An immunologic basis for these abnormalities has been described. Rats with unilaterally
ligated testes or those receiving injected homo-
genates of ischemic testes develop an increased
serum cytotoxicity with increased immunofluorescence of the contralateral nontwisted
testis. Considerable generalized cellular damage
was noted by histologic examination of these
testes [32, 33].

Ultrastructural histologic abnormalities in
the uninvolved testis of two adults who suffered
unilateral testicular torsion have been reported
[27], as well as impaired spermatogenesis in
50% of adults who had previous childhood testicular torsion [34]. Similarly, an adult follow
up of 46 men who underwent unilateral childhood orchidopexy revealed a normal semen
analysis in only 28% [35]! An additional study
revealed a 64% reduction in mean sperm
density in 29 adults having undergone previous
childhood orchidopexy for unilateral maldescent. These patients, as a group, also showed
a supranormal FSH response to LHRH stimulation [36].

These results demonstrate clearly that unilateral testicular damage can pathologically affect
the remaining normal testis. The question must
be raised, however, whether the mechanisms involved in these various conditions are one and

Table 4. Weight of descended testis of unilaterally cryptorchid 66-day-old rats

	Weight of testis	[(mg/g body wt.) × 10³]
Control (sham operated)	5.38 +	0.23
Unilateral cryptorchid	5.66 +	0.44[a]
Monorchic	7.18 +	0.55
Bilateral cryptorchid	1.73 +	0.75

[a] Not statistically significant

the same. Specifically, it must be questioned
whether the mechanism seen in cryptorchidism
is the same as in experimental immuno-orchitis
or in testicular torsion, where an immunologic
process seems operative.

In an attempt to investigate this problem further, we induced unilateral cryptorchidism in
48-h-old rats, with sham-operated, unilateral,
and bilateral castrate groups serving as references. Testicular weight, light and electron microscopy, and immunofluorescent staining of
the descended contralateral testes were done,
as well as determination of circulating antibodies and levels of FSH, LH, and testosterone.
Weights of the descended testis (Table 4) did
not differ between unilaterally cryptorchid and
sham-operated control rats. Careful light- and
electron-microscopic analysis of the descended
testes failed to reveal any differences when compared with control testes (Figs. 3–5). Circulating antibodies showed no group-specific patterns of distribution, and no immunofluorescence was seen in the descended testes of the
unilaterally cryptorchid rats. Table 5 showing
FSH, LH and testosterone levels in these
groups reveals that LH levels were elevated in
the unilaterally cryptorchid and unilaterally
castrate groups and, as expected, in the bilaterally castrate animals. Serum testosterone levels
did not differ between these groups however,
remaining in the normal range as a result of
the LH hypersecretion.

These results, in which LH elevations were
observed in the unilateral cryptorchid rats, were
not associated with any corroborative morphometric or histologic abnormalities within the
descended testis. It was not possible therefore
to demonstrate any induced effect. Similarly,
no conclusions substantiating or refuting an acquired effect on the descended testis could be
reached. In ten pubertal boys with untreated

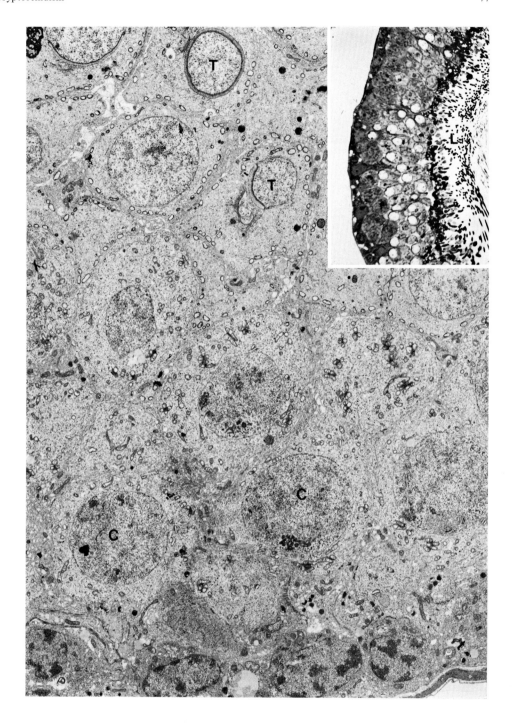

Fig. 3. Light (*inset*) and electron micrograph of testis from a 66-day-old control rat. Germ cells in various stages of spermatogenesis are present (*C*, spermatocyte; *T*, sperma- tid). Note the large number of spermatozoa in the lumen (*L*). ×3,000, inset ×800

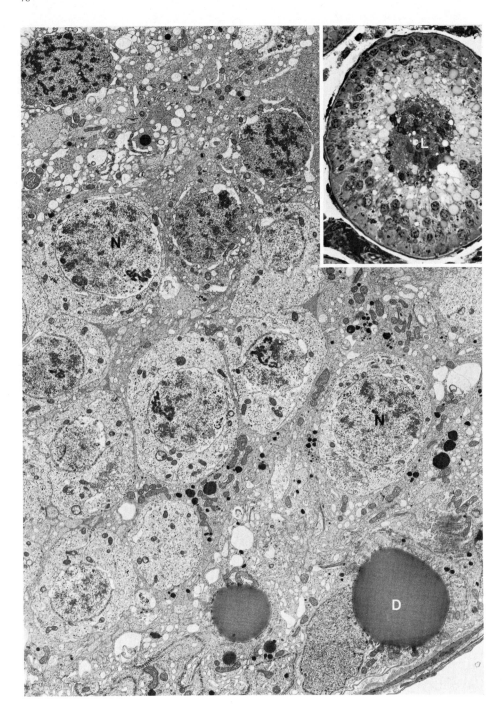

Fig. 4. Light (*inset*) and electron micrograph of a cryptorchid testis from a 66-day-old unilaterally cryptorchid rat. There is an abundance of large lipid droplets (*D*), and spermatids and spermatozoa are no longer present. The lumen (*L*) is filled with cellular debris and the spermatocyte nuclei (*N*) have many dense regions of heterochromatin which may represent early signs of degeneration. × 3,000, inset × 800

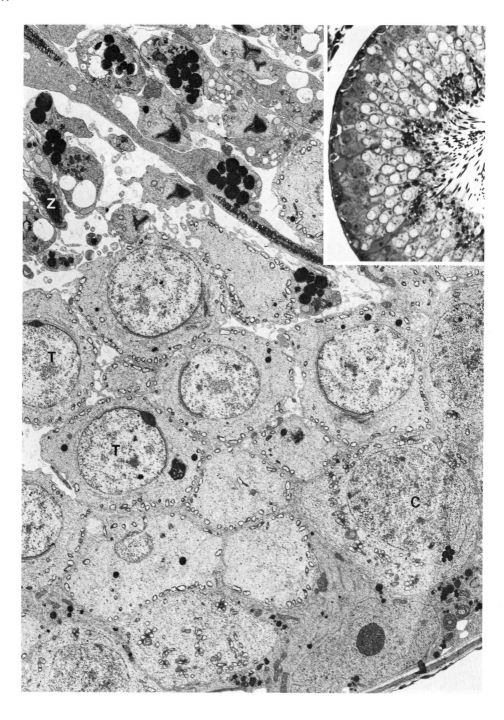

Fig. 5. Light (*inset*) and electron micrograph of the descended contralateral testis in a 66-day-old unilaterally cryptorchid rat. The descended testis appears similar to those of control animals. No signs of degeneration are evident. Spermatocytes (*C*), spermatids (*T*), and spermatozoa (*Z*) are common. × 3,000, inset × 800

Table 5. Hormonal levels in mature cryptorchid 66-day-old rats (mean $\pm$ SD)

	FSH (ng/ml)	LH (ng/ml)	Testosterone (ng/dl)
Control (sham operated)	1.84 ± 0.55	0.13 ± 0.04	254.3 ± 28
Unilateral castrate	2.11 ± 0.36	0.30 ± 0.12 ($P = 0.002$)	259.7 ± 43
Unilateral cryptorchid	2.21 ± 0.39	0.29 ± 0.08 ($P = 0.00025$)	257.1 ± 30
Bilateral cryptorchid	3.85 ± 1.89 ($P = 0.05$)	0.43 ± 0.24 ($P = 0.02$)	249.5 ± 37

(P = not significant unless indicated)

cryptorchidism, immunofluorescent staining of the undescended testis at orchiectomy failed to reveal any evidence of IgG, IgM, or C_3. In a large group of cryptorchids surveyed for circulating antisperm antibodies and for immunofluorescence of the cryptorchid and descended testes, no evidence for an immunologic process could be demonstrated [37]. These data contrast with the experimental results observed in unilateral testicular torsion, where an immunologic process appears to induce damage demonstrated by histologic examination in the normal testis. The entire question may be far more complex than it appears, in that mere testicular manipulation may be capable of induction of contralateral histologic lesions, at least on a transient basis [38]. In another preliminary investigation, 20% of adults having childhood hernia repair were found to have elevated FSH levels, in spite of normal-sized testes being present bilaterally [39]!

These studies indicate a bilateral pathologic process which may affect fertility, though they do not answer the question of its pathogenesis. One working theory conceptually unifying the various processes is that a primary congenital defect in LH secretion occurs, resulting in impairment of testicular descent, and very possibly impairment of intratesticular androgen biosynthesis as well. This process may occur in both the descended and undescended testes in unilateral cases. Subsequent damage to the undescended testis occurs by virtue of the abnormal extrascrotal position, as temperature alteration has been shown to alter intratesticular steroid conversion to testosterone. These alterations in intratesticular steroid synthesis may then affect development of the germinal epithelium and later affect spermatogenesis. The histologic and hormonal abnormalities cited in this chapter and in this book are compatible with the occurrence of an early defect of this nature, and of hormonal "understimulation," and offer the rationale for early treatment and perhaps hormonal supplementation therapy thereafter.

An alternative theory explaining the observed impairment of fertility seen in unilateral cryptorchidism requires that an induced secondary (immunologic) insult occurs in the descended testis, as appears to occur in unilateral testicular torsion. Evidence of this nature to date has not been conclusive.

Acknowledgments. I am grateful for the continued stimulation and collaboration provided by my associates, Drs. Selwyn B. Levitt and Paul Smey of the Division of Pediatric Urology, and by Dr. Boyce Bennett of the Department of Pathology, The Albert Einstein College of Medicine; and by Drs. Bernard Gondos and Eric Sun of the Department of Pathology, University of Connecticut, School of Medicine. The assistance in the preparation of this manuscript by my secretarial staff, Edna Marash, Mary Scheffer, Marie D'Alo, Kathleen Maguire, and Cynthia Chiavelli, is similarly appreciated and acknowledged.

References

1. Charny CW (1960) The spermatogenic potential of the undescended testis before and after treatment. J Urol 83:697

2. Bergada C, Farias ME, Romero de Behar BM, Cullen M (1969) Abnormal sex chromatin pattern in cryptorchidism, girls with short stature and other endocrine patients. Helv Paediatr Acta 4:372

3. Ludwig G, Potempa J (1973) Der optimale Zeitpunkt der Behandlung des Kryptorchismus. Deutsch Med Wochenschr 100:680

4. Giarola A, Agostini G (1979) Undescended testis and male fertility. In: Bierich JR, Giarola A (eds) Cryptorchidism. Academic Press, London New York, p 533

5. Puri P, Nixon HH (1977) Bilateral retractile testes – subsequent effects on fertility. J Pediatr Surg 12:563

6. Illig R, Exner GU, Killmann F, Kellerer K, Borkenstein M, Lunglmayr L, Kuber W, Prader A (1977) Treatment of cryptorchidism by intravasal synthetic luteinizing-hormone releasing treatment. Lancet 2:518

7. Fahlstrom G, Helmberg L, Johansson H (1960) Atrophy of the testes following operations upon the inguinal region in infants and children. Acta Chir Scand 126:221

8. Mengel W, Hecker WC, Moritz P (1977) The treatment of the maldescended testis under special consideration of the moment of surgical treatment. In: Bierich JR, Rager K, Ranke MB (eds) Maldescensus testis. Urban & Schwarzenberg, München Baltimore, p 111

9. Gross RE, Replogle RL (1963) Treatment of the undescended testis. Postgrad Med 34:266

10. Sherins RJ, Brightwell D, Sternthal PM (1977) Longitudinal analysis of semen of fertile and infertile men. In: Nankin HR, Troen P (eds) The testis in normal and infertile men. Raven Press, New York

11. Knorr W, Proschold U, Richter W (1976) Fertility after treatment of maldescensus testis. In: Bierich JR, Rager K, Ranke MB (eds) Maldescensus testis. Urban & Schwarzenberg, München Baltimore, p 95

12. Freund M (1966) Standards for the rating of human sperm morphology: a cooperative study. Int J Fertil 11:97

13. Gross RE, Jewett TC Jr (1956) Surgical experience from 1,222 operations for undescended testes. JAMA 160:634

14. WHO (World Health Organization) Statistics, Geneva, 1969

15. Zamudio-Albescu J (1979) Cryptorchidism and fertility. In: Bierich JR, Giarola A (eds) Cryptorchidism. Academic Press, London New York, p 497

16. Bergada C (1979) Use of gonadotropins for the evaluation of testicular function and correlations to biopsy of cryptorchid testes. In: Job JC (ed) Cryptorchidism: diagnosis and treatment. Karger, Basel New York (Pediatric and adolescent endocrinology, vol 6, p 97)

17. Richter W, Proschold M, Butenandt O, Knorr D (1976) Die Fertilität nach HCG-Behandlung des Maldescensus testis. Klin Wochenschr 54:467–473

18. Bierich JR (1981) Gonadotropin therapy for the undescended testis. In: Kogan SJ, Hafez ESE (eds) Pediatric andrology. Martinus Nijhoff, The Hague (Clinics in andrology, vol 7, p 163)

19. Tato L, Mase R, Rossignoli R, Pinelli L, Gaburro D (1979) Some semiological aspects of cryptorchidism in prepubertal boys: testicular volume and gonadotropin responses to LH-RH. In: Bierich JR, Giarola J (eds) Cryptorchidism. Academic Press, London New York, p 337

20. Laron Z, Dickerman Z, Ritterman I (1979) Compensatory testicular hypertrophy in unilateral cryptorchidism. In: Job JC (ed) Cryptorchidism: diagnosis and treatment. Karger, Basel New York (Pediatric and adolescent endocrinology, vol 6, p 137)

21. Kogan SJ, Smey P, Levitt SB (1979) Unpublished data

22. Hecker WC, Heinz HA (1967) Cryptorchidism and fertility. J Pediatr Surg 2:513

23. Mengel W, Heinz HA, Sippe WG (1974) Studies on cryptorchidism: a comparison of histologic findings in the germinative epithelium before and after the second year of life. J Pediatr Surg 9:445

24. Hedinger C (1977) The histopathology of the cryptorchid testis. In: Bierich JR, Rager K, Ranke MB (eds) Maldescensus testis. Urban & Schwarzenberg, München Baltimore, p 29

25. Brown PC, Dorling J, Glynn LE (1972) Ultrastructural changes in experimental allergic orchitis in guinea pigs. J Pathol 106:229

26. Tung KSK, Alexander NJ (1977) Autoimmune reactions in the testis. In: Johnson AD, Gomes WR (eds) The testis, vol IV. Academic Press, London New York, p 491

27. Chakraborty J, Jhonjhunwala J, Nelson L, Young M (1980) Effects of unilateral torsion of the spermatic cord on the contralateral testis in human and guinea pig. Arch Androl 4:95

28. Shirai M, Matsushita S, Kagayama M (1966) Histologic changes of the scrotal testis in unilateral cryptorchidism. Tohoku J Exp Med 90:363

29. Weissbach L, Ibach B (1977) Morphometrical studies on experimental unilateral cryptorchids in the dog. In: Bierich JR, Rager K, Ranke MB (eds) Maldescensus testis. Urban & Schwarzenberg, München Baltimore, p 165

30. Mengel W, Moritz P, Huttmann B (1979) Experimental studies on pathogenesis of the histological changes in unilateral cryptorchidism. In: Bierich JR, Giarola A (eds) Cryptorchidism. Academic Press, London New York, p 135

31. Katz S (to be published) Assessment of fertility after testicular torsion: an experimental study. Invest Urol

32. Harrison RG, Lewis-Jones DI, Moreno de Marval MJ, Connolly RC (1981) Mechanism of damage to the contralateral testis in rats with an ischaemic testis. Preliminary communication. Lancet 2:723

33. Wallace DMA, Hendry WF, Gunter PA, Landon GV, Pugh RCB (1981) Sympathetic orchiopathia. Lancet 2:1173

34. Bartsch G, Frank S, Mikuz G, Marberger H (1980) Late results in testicular torsion with special regards to fertility and endocrinology. J Urol 124:375

35. Scheiber K, Menardi G, Marberger H, Bartsch G (1981) Late results after surgical tratment of maldescended testes with special regard to exocrine and endocrine testicular function. Eur Urol 7:268

36. Lipschultz LI, Caminos-Torres R, Greenspan CS, Snyder PJ (1976) Testicular function after orchidopexy for unilaterally undescended testes. N Engl J Med 295:15

37. Isidori A, Dondero F, Spera G (1979) Immunological

studies in cryptorchidism. In: Bierich JR, Giarola A (eds) Cryptorchidism. Academic Press, London New York, p 207

38. Frankenhuis MT, Wensing CJG (1979) Induction of spermatogenesis in the naturally cryptorchid pig. Fertil Steril 31:428–433
39. Laron Z (1981) Personal communication
40. Madersbacher H, Kövesdi S, Frick J (1972) Zur Fertilität beim einseitigen Kryptorchismus. Urologie 11: 210–212
41. Schreiber G, Schickedanz H, Sellen B (1976) Morphologische und biochemische Spermiogrammbefunde nach chirurgisch behandeltem Maldeszensus testis. Z Urol 69:667–671
42. Werder EA, Illig R, Torresoni T, Zachmann M, Bauman P, Ott F, Prader A (1976) Gonadal function in young adults after surgical treatment of cryptorchidism. Br Med J 2:1357–1359

43. Lipschultz LI, Ceminos-Torres R, Greenspon CS (1976) Testicular function after orchidopexy for unilateral undescended testis. N Engl J Med 295:15–17
44. Retief PJM (1977) Fertility in undescended testes. S Afr Med J 52:610–
45. Wojciechowski K, Rucki T, Walczak M, Syc AK (1977) Longterm results of undescended testicle operative treatment. Prog Pediatr Surg 10:297–304
46. Knorr D (1979) Fertility after HCG-treatment of maldescended testes. In: Job JC (ed) Cryptorchidism. Diagnosis and treatment. Karger, Basel
47. Czeplicki P (1975) Actualités gynécologiques No. 6:177–189
48. Bramble F, Houghton AL, Eccles S, O'Shea A, Jacobs HS (1974) Reproductive and endocrine function after surgical treatment of bilateral cryptorchidism. Lancet 2:311–314

7 Cryptorchidism and Malignant Testicular Disease

W.J. Cromie

The term cryptorchidism is derived from two Greek words – *kryptos,* meaning hidden, and *orchis,* denoting testicle. – Hidden within this testis is the propensity to develop neoplasia. In this chapter the theoretical, environmental, physical, and histologic factors that interact to produce malignant disease in the testis of the cryptorchid male will be discussed.

7.1 Etiologic Theories of Malignant Degeneration

Various theories have been postulated to explain malignant degeneration of the undescended testis (Table 1). Fergusson noted a history of trauma in 10% of patients with a malignant testis [1]. This correlation with trauma is most likely attributable to the fact that medical attention was promptly sought as a result of the minor trauma, which then led to the discovery of the testicular tumor, rather than any suspicion of neoplasm from trauma. If trauma was indeed a significant precipitating factor, one would expect a lower incidence of tumor in well-protected, intra-abdominal undescended testes than in scrotal testes. In fact, the opposite is true. The one circumstance in which trauma may play a role is when significant testicular injury results in subsequent atrophy. Another theory, according to which altered environment adversely affects the developing seminiferous tubules, has been suggested by Kaufman and Bruce [2]. Germinal atrophy and chronic temperature elevation have been implicated by others [3, 4, 5].

In 1962, Wershub suggested that some form of hormonal imbalance was responsible for testicular histologic changes [6], and recently Hadžiselimović and Girard lent further support to this theory. They proposed that a suppression of endocrine gonadal function of the hypothalamus and pituitary gland occurred during intrauterine development in affected males [7]. This would not only adversely affect the Leydig cells, but could also produce some form of germ cell defect, as proposed by Sohval [8]. From a retrospective viewpoint, it appears that all of these etiologic factors may be interrelated and cumulative in their adverse effect on testicular development. For the sake of completeness and clarification, it would be worthwhile to consider additional factors that collectively place the male population at risk of developing testicular tumors.

7.2 General Risk Factors in Testicular Cancer (Table 2)

Characteristically, the peak incidence of testicular cancer occurs between the ages of 25 and 35 years. This is followed by a decline and a subsequent rise in incidence after the age of 65 years. During the past several decades, mortality in patients with testicular cancer has gradually increased in Caucasian American males aged 15 to 29 years, while simultaneously falling in older white males. The age-adjusted incidence in African and Oriental populations is considerably lower than that in American and European whites, and is persistently lower in blacks. The reasons for this racial variation remains obscure [9].

Table 1. Etiology of malignancy in cryptorchidism

Etiology	Authors
Trauma	Fergusson [1]
Altered environment	Kaufman and Bruce [2]
Temperature elevation	Mostofi [3, 4]
Germinal atrophy	Hausfeld [5]
Hormonal imbalance	Wershub [6]
Inherent germinal cell defect	Sohval [8]

Table 2. Risk factors for testicular malignancy

Factor	Authors
Race and socioeconomic group	Graham and Gibson [10]
Location of testis	Campbell [11]
Hernia and GU anomalies	Li and Fraumeni [13]
Age at cryptorchid repair	Kiesewetter et al. [14]
Estrogen exposure in utero	Gill et al. [15]
HLA-Dw7 antigen	DeWolf et al. [18]
Maternal pelvic and abdominal radiation	Henderson et al. [9]
Jockey shorts	Loughlin et al. [19]
Mumps	Kaufman and Bruce [2]
Atrophy, infertility, and cancer in situ	Skakkebaek and Berthelsen [29]

The incidence of testicular cancer doubled from 1938 to 1975. Again, the greatest increase occurred in younger men. In a social epidemiologic survey of 247 patients with testicular cancer, Graham and Gibson discovered some interesting differences in demographic parameters and risk of testicular cancer between these patients and 2,504 control subjects [10]. In their survey population, they discovered an increased risk of testicular cancer in inhabitants of small towns compared with those from large cities, in professionals as compared with other occupational groups, in Protestants compared with Catholics, and in native-born Americans as compared with foreign-born immigrants.

Location of the testis has always had a significant bearing on the incidence of malignant disease. Campbell was the first to document this influence. He reported a sixfold increase in the risk of testicular tumor when the testis was situated within the abdomen, as compared to when it was in the lower inguinal or higher scrotal regions [11]. While there are differences of opinion as to the actual increase in risk, there is no question that an intra-abdominal testis is associated with a higher incidence of neoplasia than a testis situated elsewhere [12]. Li and Fraumeni noted an increased incidence of testicular tumors in children with hernias, cryptorchidism, and other genitourinary anomalies, suggesting that neoplasia and genitourinary anomalies share prenatal determinants for the subsequent development of neoplasia [13]. Conversely, Kieswetter has suggested that early successful repair of cryptorchidism decreases the risk of germinal atrophy, thus somewhat diminishing the risk of testicular cancer [14].

Henderson has proposed that histologic changes occur in the cryptorchid testis as a result of excessive amounts of free estrogen or progesterone that are present during the first trimester of pregnancy [9]. He supports this hypothesis with the observation that in utero exposure to exogenous estrogens in the form of diethylstilbestrol (DES) and oral contraceptives can lead to cryptorchidism. Gill et al. studied 300 men who were exposed to DES in utero and found that 26 had testicular hypoplasia. Seventeen of the 26 had cryptorchidism, further substantiating this observation [15]. Similar effects have been reported in the male offspring of pregnant animals given DES. The etiology of nausea in pregnancy is not completely understood, but nausea is a common side effect of exogenous estrogen administration, and nausea in pregnancy may similarly be due to temporary high levels of free estrogen. In a recent case control study, Henderson found a correlation between excessive nausea, vomiting, and exogenous hormone used during the index pregnancy and subsequent testicular cancer. Thus cryptorchidism and excessive nausea, together with the use of hormones, may be combined into a single hypothesis that a major risk factor for testicular cancer is the presence of an excess of estrogen at the time of testicular differentiation.

Although exogenous exposure to estrogen may have some effect, information from a Hungarian study suggests the involvement of hormonal factors – in this case, hormones that are endogenously produced. Czeizel et al. found in an epidemiologic survey of 689 neonates with undescended testes that seasonal distribution of undescended testes at birth was significant [16, 17]. Between March and May (with a maximum incidence in March), a significantly greater number of boys were born with undescended testes. Conversely, the occurrence was considerably lower in those born between August and December (with a minimal incidence in October) [16]. His rationale for this difference cited the seasonal changes in the production of pituitary gonadotropins, depending on the duration of daylight. The shortest and longest days of the year are December 23rd and June 23rd respectively, and the observed maximal and minimal incidences of true undescended testes occurred 2–4 months later. As a corollary to this study, the mothers of cryptorchid boys in the index population were reviewed and were found to have had a later onset of menarche and significantly shorter menses than did the control population. In 21.2% of the mothers of patients with undescended testes, menarche commenced after the age of 15 years. Only 10.9% of the mothers of the controls experienced this late onset. It is suggested, then, that mild pituitary hypogonadism of mothers may be a predisposing factor for undescended testes in their sons [17].

Human leukocyte antigen (HLA) is involved not only in transplantation, but also in many diseased states. DeWolf et al. recently revealed tissue-typing results from a group of patients with testicular cancer [18]. The results showed an abnormally high antigen frequency for HLA-Dw7 in patients with testicular teratocarcinoma. The biological significance of this finding, as well as the associations of other diseases with HLA, is unknown. However, four possible mechanisms have been suggested. First, HLA antigens may cross-react with pathogenic antigens, leading to cross-tolerance. The pathogen, then, would not be subjected to the host immune mechanisms. Second, HLA antigens may function as surface cell receptors for particular pathogens, similar to the association between malaria and susceptible red cells. Third, there may be genetic linkage between genes controlling the expression of HLA and genes controlling the immune responsiveness of the host. Likewise, HLA antigens may serve as markers for specific genes, causing deficiencies in specific normal proteins that affect the levels of the second and fourth components of complement. Whatever mechanisms apply, the association between HLA and testicular teratocarcinoma has implicated heredity as a possible etiologic factor in the development of testicular cancer. This is of particular interest in view of the fact that at least 18 cases of familial testicular cancer have been reported [18].

Other risk factors may also contribute to the occurrence of testicular cancer. In a pilot case control study of the risk factors associated with this type of cancer, Loughlin et al. revealed an increased risk in males whose mothers underwent abdominal or pelvic radiography during pregnancy. Of additional interest was a positive association between testicular cancer and the use of jockey undershorts as compared with boxer undershorts. The suggested mechanism was thought to be the increased testicular temperature associated with jockey shorts [19]. Finally, some evidence suggests an association between mumps orchitis and testicular cancer, particularly in those patients with associated atrophy [2].

From this brief overview, it becomes apparent that multiple factors may contribute to the development of testicular neoplasia. In some cases, these factors may be both the cause and the effect of cryptorchidism abnormalities. In others, these factors contribute an added risk to an already compromised gonad.

Consideration of the relationship between testicular neoplasia and cryptorchidism becomes particularly germane when considering the contralateral scrotal testis. It may well be that the ultimate adverse effect of the risk factors mentioned involves the germinal cell line of both developing gonads. For lack of a better term, let us presume that some degree of dysgenesis occurs. If this is the case, then a direct correlation may exist between the development of dysgenesis and the development of malignant disease of the testis. Sohval has noted a greatly increased incidence of dysgenetic tissue in cryptorchid testes, and suggests that this may account for the relative vulnerability of the testes to malignant degeneration [8]. If dysgenesis is a factor in testicular tumorigenesis, then the field change effect in the contralateral scrotal testis will likely be adverse as well. It is not surprising that an increased incidence of neoplasia in the descended testis has been reported in patients with unilateral cryptorchidism [20, 21, 22]. By way of example, Johnson reported that one of five cryptorchid patients with a testicular tumor also developed a tumor in the contralateral testis [23]. From a review of the literature, he also suggested that patients with unilateral cryptorchidism had a 15% chance of developing a tumor in the opposite testis if one testis was already involved with tumor. Of those patients with bilateral cryptorchidism and testicular tumor, 25% will develop neoplasia in both gonads. In light of this fact, it would be worthwhile to consider the histologic characteristics of the cryptorchid testis that may result in vulnerability to malignant neoplasia.

7.3 Premalignant Histologic Changes in the Cryptorchid Gonad

A brief summary of the known histologic findings in the cryptorchid gonad is warranted, as is a discussion of some of the implications of in situ change, with specific emphasis on the atrophic testis.

Histologic changes within the cryptorchid gonad have been well documented by Hadziselimovic [24], and this report confirms the work of others [4, 14, 25]. He discovered that Leydig cell atrophy could be documented in the neonate (see also Chapt. 4). By the time the patient was 2 years of age, an increase in peritubular connective tissue was evident, as was early spermatogonial atrophy. By late childhood or early adolescence more dramatic changes were apparent, such as a decreased number of spermatogonia, diminution of seminiferous tubular diameter, and decreased or absent spermatogenesis. It has also been documented that the magnitude of histologic change increases as the testis becomes more abdominal in position [14]. Until recently, the clinician could not detect which testis in this large subgroup would ultimately undergo malignant change, despite this information. Recently, Skakkebaek and his colleagues identified a possible premalignant change in the tubular epithelium that provides a glimmer of hope for detection of the individual at risk [26]. They have characterized the findings as germ cell tumor in situ and have described their findings. Large and atypical germ cells with higher than normal DNA content are present along with seminiferous tubules with early germinal elements such as gonocytes and prespermatogonia. In some cases occasional mitotic activity is seen, with some seminiferous tubular cells located outside the walls of the tubule. Waxman [27] of the United States and Nuesch-Bachmann [28] of Switzerland, have found similar abnormalities in surveys of infertile men with atrophic gonads. This is powerful evidence that the atypical appearances of the germ cells are premalignant and that the condition may justifiable be classified as carcinoma in situ. It also appears that these histologic abnormalities are sufficiently widespread in the testis to be detected by a random biopsy[1]. Skakkebaek and his group went even further, identifying four groups of men who are "at risk" of developing tumor. The first group in-

cludes men presenting with infertility who are found to have small, atrophic testes [26]. The second group is composed of men who have previously undergone orchidopexy and who have a small testis [29]. The third includes patients who have already had a germ cell tumor diagnosed in one testis and who demonstrate similar histologic findings in the contralateral testis. Finally, these histologic characteristics have been found in the abnormal gonads of individuals with testicular feminization syndrome [30]. Thus in patients with undescended testes, this extra risk appears to affect the testis even after orchidopexy, although the recent trend toward early correction in childhood may reduce the incidence of these adverse effects [14]. Atypical germ cells have occasionally been described in patients with cryptorchid testes [27], but Krabbe et al. discovered carcinoma in situ in 4 of 50 men previously treated for undescended testes [31]. Two of these patients had an unsuspected, invasive tumor in the adjacent testicular tissue. In all four patients the contralateral testis was normal, whereas the affected testis was small and atrophic in three cases [32]. It would appear to be of more than passing significance that in three, and possibly all four, of Skakkebaek's categories the gonads affected with carcinoma in situ were atrophic for varied reasons.

The role of testicular atrophy as a causal factor in tumorigenesis has been the subject of considerable conjecture; however, little clinical or experimental data has been recorded [33, 34]. One of the obvious problems is the detection of a prior history of atrophy in an individual with testicular tumor. Nonetheless, the cumulative data of Skakkebaek adds much to Kaufman and Bruce's observations of seminoma in an atrophic testis following mumps orchitis [2]. Review of the pathologic sections revealed that the tumor developed in juxtaposition to the atrophic tubules. They suggested that the nature of atrophy is probably less important than the mere presence of atrophy. This observation is further confirmed by experimentally produced testicular tumors in animals. Carleton et al. observed that atypical cells were first seen adjacent to the damaged tissue as early as 1 week after injection of zinc [35]. Frank neoplasms occurred 10 weeks after the injection and were monocellular, similar to seminomatous and embryonal carcinoma in man. After 3 months, a teratoid differentiation developed which appeared to be derived from the monocellular tumor. The investigators observed that zinc or heavy metals were not involved directly in teratogenesis, but produced tumor only insofar as they produced tissue necrosis.

The histologic changes within the cryptorchid gonad, therefore, may be affected by the etiologic mechanism responsible for maldescent as well as by all of the previously enumerated risk factors for developing neoplasia. The factor that causes atrophy, whether it be maldescent, anoxia (in the case of testicular torsion), histotoxin (in mumps orchitis), or chemical toxin (in metal-induced experimental tumors), may be the final common pathway toward an understanding of tumorigenesis.

7.4 Tumor Cell Types in Undescended Testes

It has long been purported that the distribution of germinal cell tumors in undescended testes is somewhat different than that occurring in scrotal testes. Pugh and Collins suggested that seminoma comprised 60% of the tumors occurring in undescended testes, compared with 30%–40% of the germ cell tumors occurring in scrotal testes [36]. Similarly, a slight increase in the incidence of teratomas and teratocarcinomas was noted. Recently, Martin reviewed 167 patients with tumor after orchidopexy in whom cell type was precisely reported [12]. He combined this data with Batata's review of 83 such patients at New York Memorial Hospital [37]. Combined incidence figures are detailed in Table 3, revealing a cell pattern in post-orchidopexy tumors that is quite similar to that found in patients with normally descended testes. The increased incidence of nonseminomatous tumors portends a less favorable prognosis for these patients; it also clearly underscores the fact that seminoma does not occur with the frequency that was previously suggested.

In addition to the research on the cell types of postorchidopexy testicular tumors, there is other noteworthy data regarding the behavior of these neoplasms. Of 1,000 patients treated at Sloan-Kettering for testicular tumors, 125 (12.5%) had a previous history of cryptorchi-

Table 3. Tumors after orchiopexy

	n	%
Seminoma	58	34
Embryonal cell Ca including other elements	53	32
Teratocarcinoma including other elements	53	32
Choriocarcinoma	3	2
	167	100

dism. Eighty-three patients had descended testes. In 21 patients the testis descended spontaneously, 51 required orchidopexy, and 11 underwent hormonal therapy. Forty-two patients with uncorrected undescended testes served as controls. In all patients, the median age at which orchidopexy was performed was 12 years. This procedure did not appear to be helpful in preventing malignant disease, nor did it affect the time of tumor occurrence, as 32 years was the median age at which neoplasia occurred for both corrected and uncorrected patients. Thus orchidopexy – at 12 years of age or later – clearly does not influence the natural history of neoplastic development [37]. In a review of the literature, Martin noted that in only six patients did germinal cell tumor develop if orchidopexy had been performed prior to 8 years of age [12]. This observation suggests that early orchidopexy may be associated with a decreased risk of subsequent tumor formation.

On a further review of Batata's data, it was noted that the tumor stage at diagnosis was similar for corrected and uncorrected cases and that there appeared to be little effect on the development of distant metastasis for stage I and stage II tumors. The 5-year survival rate for corrected vs uncorrected cryptorchid patients was almost identical, with a slight increase in survival of the surgically corrected patients with nonseminomatous tumors. The 5-year survival rate also appeared to be unaffected by the location of the gonad, as there was 60% survival whether the testis was found in the scrotum, the groin, or the abdomen. In the final analysis of this series, the prognosis in cryptorchid patients with testicular cancer was determined by the histologic grade and anatomic stage of the tumor, not by the location of the testis or any previous form of correction. The survival for stage I tumors was 87%; for stage II tumors 41%; and for stage III tumors 26%. The overall 5-year survival rate is almost identical to that of patients with testicular tumors affecting normal scrotal testes.

7.5 Incidence and Risk Analysis of Malignant Disease with Cryptorchidism

There is no question that cryptorchidism places the affected patient at increased risk of subsequent development of a testicular tumor. However, this risk must be considered in relationship to both the incidence of all malignant neoplasms of the testis occurring in the general population and the incidence of mortality associated with other malignant processes in the male.

Testicular tumors are rare, and the increased danger of malignant disease can only be determined if the population at risk is clearly defined. Interpretation of incidence rates is made difficult, however, by the uncertainty of older sources of information, the small numbers of patients involved in recent observations, and the lack of knowledge regarding the size of the source population. This difficulty is further compounded in the relationship of the cryptorchid testis to the subsequent risk of malignant disease and by the interval between surgical repair and the occurrence of a secondary neoplasm. Martin and Whitaker attempted to bring some order to risk assessment by pooling collected series [12, 38]. They found that 9.8% of all germ cell tumors arise in cryptorchid testes. Using Campbell's extensive survey of European and American military recruits, the incidence of cryptorchidism was found to be 0.28%. If this figure is accepted, a multiple of 35 would be required to raise this small group at risk to the observed incidence of 9.8% ($0.28 \times 35 = 9.8$) [39]. This view has been corroborated by several other authors, who show the probability of malignant disease in an undescended testis as 20–40 times greater than that of the normally located scrotal testis [11, 22]. It must be borne in mind that this represents a combined risk for all cryptorchid males, regardless of the location of the gonad. Campbell also found that whereas most undescended testes were located in the low inguinal region, 14.5% of those located intra-abdominally were

responsible for 48.5% of the testes involved with malignant tumor [11]. Thus, although the intra-abdominal undescended testis is less common, it has a fourfold greater chance of developing a malignant neoplasm than testes in other locations.

Recently Cromie and Sedransk derived a mathematical formula based on available information on the occurrence of testicular malignant disease in the normal population, incidence of cryptorchidism, and notations of a history of cryptorchidism in selected patients with testicular tumors [40]. Using a Bayesian approach and Poisson processes, values were found to express both an estimate and an uncertainty of the risk of testicular tumors consequent to cryptorchidism. A single value determined for the risk of malignant disease in patients with cryptorchidism was 48.91 per 100,000, which represents a 22.23-fold increase compared with the risk in those individuals with scrotal testes, in whom the incidence of malignant neoplasm was 2.2 per 100,000. The major problem with these data is the inability of the average clinician to relate them to morbidity or mortality consequent to tumor occurrence. To better conceptualize this information, we used the standard method of reporting tumor occurrence, incidence per 100,000, to compare the incidence of testicular tumors with other malignant diseases (Fig. 1). Using the incidence rate of 48 per 100,000 for testicular tumor in patients with cryptorchidism, the chance of developing colorectal, prostatic, lung, or gastrointestinal tumors is greater. Conversely, tumors of the brain and oral cavity, as well as childhood and hematologic neoplasms, when combined, have a lesser incidence. Testicular tumors in adults, on the far left of the graph, represent 2.2 per 100,000 population. To take this process one step further, inguinal and abdominal undescended testes were differentiated (Fig. 2), indicating a diminished risk in inguinal cryptorchidism and a fourfold increased risk for the patient with abdominal cryptorchidism. When comparing this risk with that of other malignant diseases that occur in the adult, such as prostatic carcinoma, the risk is doubled in the patient with an intra-abdominal testis. Although there is no question that an intra-abdominal undescended testis increases the risk of testicular tumors in individuals, given the best forms of therapy what is the chance of

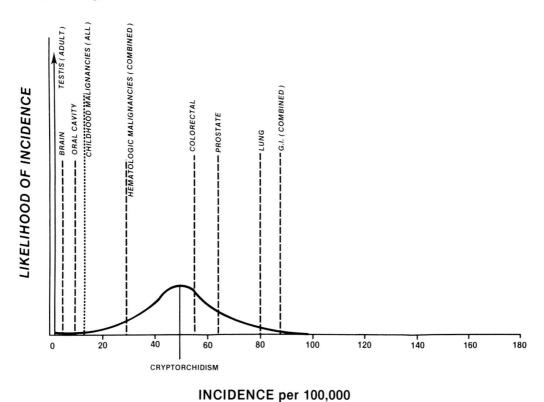

Fig. 1. Comparison of incidence of malignancies with incidence of testicular tumors in cryptorchidism

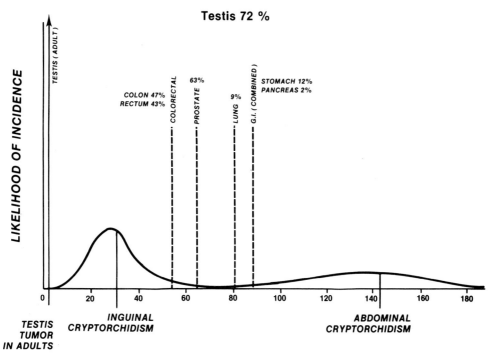

Fig. 2. Relative 5-year survival rates of testis and other adult neoplasms. (Myers and Hankey [41])

5-year survival? The percentages of 5-year survival rates for several neoplasms are listed in Fig. 2. Testicular tumor, regardless of cell type or stage at presentation, had an overall 5-year survival rate of 72% when this survey was completed in 1973 and subsequently published in 1980 by the National Institutes of Health [41]. With the improvements in evaluation and management of patients with testicular tumors, it is clear that the occurrence of a testicular neoplasm is not necessarily a death sentence. In fact with adjuvant chemotherapy programs, using *cis*-platinum, vinblastine, and bleomycin, with or without associated retroperitoneal lymphadenectomy, impressive response and survival rates are being reported. Currently, it is generally accepted that the "long-term cure rates of patients with metastatic testicular cancer treated with intensive combination chemotherapy is in the range of 80–90%, although the prognosis for any one individual is most closely related to the extent of disease at the time of treatment" [42]. It is also likely that low-dose, graded-adjuvant, chemotherapeutic regimens appropriate to the risk of recurrence within each pathologic stage will be considered, instead of observation followed by intensive chemotherapy at tumor relapse. In summary, in addressing the issue of malignant risk in the undescended testis, we may well be discussing not the prospect of future mortality, but a transient episode of morbidity as a result of chemotherapy.

7.6 Theoretical Considerations

It is clear that cryptorchidism increases the risk of subsequent testicular neoplasm, but many questions regarding the mechanism of neoplastic transformation remain. Is the testis predisposed to malignant disease as a result of events occurring in utero, or do subsequent relocation and therapeutic endeavors at various ages alter this course? It is also important to determine what factors place the gonad at increased risk and what factors are responsible for the occurrence of neoplasia in the normally descended contralateral testis. From the data reviewed in this chapter, it appears that testicular location and correction of the cryptorchid gonad after 12 years of age does not alter tumor occurrence. Only time will tell if earlier orchidopexy will affect these observations.

Considering all these variables, is it possible to describe the events that precipitate the transition from cryptorchid to malignant testis? I would like to submit the following scheme (Fig. 3). Through a combination of endogenous and exogenous events, a disruption of the hypo-

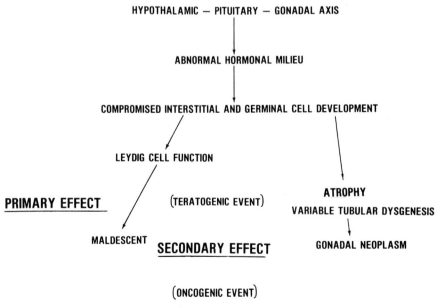

Fig. 3. Theory of development of malignancy

thalamic-pituitary-gonadal axis occurs. This results in an abnormal hormonal milieu that affects the development of the gonadal ridge, the wolffian duct structures of the mesonephros, and the gubernacular mesenchyme. The cumulative effect is an alteration in the number and character of the interstitial and germ cell lines. The primary effect may be manifested in utero in impaired Leydig cell function with diminished production of testosterone, resulting in abnormal epididymal and gubernacular development. The visible manifestation of this hormonal imbalance is testicular maldescent.

The effect on the germinal cell line is much more insidious and is subject to many more variables. The multiple factors that affect germ cell development may result in various degrees of atrophy and tubular dysgenesis. Compounding this are the risk factors previously discussed that further alter seminiferous tubular morphology. This sequence of events is similar to the two-hit theory of teratogenesis and oncogenesis proposed by Knudson and Strong [43]. According to this theory, the first stage, or teratogenic event, produces germinal mutation prenatally, resulting in a congenital anomaly – in our case, an undescended testis. This creates a substrate for the second, "post-natal event," which is carcinogenic and is aggravated by agents that are responsible for the production of atrophy. While this theory was initially developed for Wilms' tumor, it has long been thought that teratogenesis and oncogenesis represent different developmental stages of a reaction to the same injurious event. The enigma that remains hidden within the cryptorchid testis intersects this concept in some way. It remains a continuing challenge to individuals interested in cryptorchidism to bring further order, knowledge, and understanding to this "cascade to malignancy."

References

1. Fergusson JD (1962) Tumors of the testis. Br J Urol 34:407
2. Kaufman JJ, Bruce PT (1963) Testicular atrophy following mumps: a cause of testis tumor? Br J Urol 35:67
3. Ashley DJB, Mostofi FK (1959) The spermatogenic function of tumorbearing testes. J Urol 81:773
4. Dow JA, Mostofi FK (1967) Testicular tumors following orchiopexy. South Med J 60:193
5. Hausfeld KF, Schrandt D (1965) Malignancy of the testis following atrophy. J Urol 94:69
6. Wershub CP (1962) The human testis: A clinical treatise. Thomas, Springfield
7. Hadžiselimović F, Girard J (1977) Pathogenesis of cryptorchidism. Horm Res 8:76–83
8. Sohval AR (1954) Histopathology of cryptorchidism. Am J Med 16:346
9. Henderson BE, et al. (1979) Risk factors for cancer of the testis in young men. Int J Cancer 23:598–602
10. Graham S, Gibson RW (1972) Social epidemiology of cancer of the testis. Cancer 29:1242
11. Campbell HE (1942) Incidence of malignant growth of the undescended testis. Arch Surg 44:353
12. Martin DC (1979) Germinal cell tumors of the testis after orchiopexy. J Urol 121:422
13. Li F, Fraumeni JF (1972) Testicular cancer in children: epidemiologic characteristics. J Natl Cancer Inst 48; No. 6, 1575
14. Kiesewetter WB et al. (1969) Histologic changes in the testis following anatomically successful orchiopexy. J Pediatr Surg 4:59
15. Gill WB et al. (1979) Association of DES exposure in utero with cryptorchidism, testicular hypoplasia and semen abnormalities. J Urol 122:36
16. Czeizel A et al. (1981) An epidemiological study of undescended testis. J Urol 126:524
17. Czeizel A et al. (1981) Genetics of undescended testis. J Urol 126:528
18. DeWolf WC et al. (1979) HLA and testicular cancer. Nature 277:216–217
19. Loughlin JE et al. (1980) Risk factors for cancer of the testis. N Engl J Med 303:112
20. Campbell HE (1959) The incidence of malignant growth of the undescended testicle: A reply and re-evaluation. J Urol 81:663
21. Schwartz JW, Reed JF Jr (1956) The pathology of cryptorchidism. J Urol 76:429
22. Thurzo R, Pinter J (1961) Cryptorchidism and malignancy in men and animals. Urol Int 11:216
23. Johnson DC, Woodhead DM, Pohl DR (1968) Cryptorchidism and testicular tumorgenesis. Surgery 63:919
24. Hadžiselimović F (1977) Cryptorchidism: Ultrastructure of normal and cryptorchid testis. Adv Anat Embryol Cell Biol 53/3 10–65
25. Sohval AR (1954) Testicular dysgenesis as an etiologic factor in cryptorchidism. J Urol 72:693
26. Skakkebaek NE (1972) Possible carcinoma in-situ of the testis. Lancet 2:516
27. Waxman M (1976) Malignant germ cell tumor in situ in a cryptorchid testis. Cancer 38:1452–1456
28. Nuesch-Bachmann IH, Hedinger C (1977) Atypische Spermatogonien als Präkanzerose. Schweiz Med Wochenschr 107:795–801
29. Skakkebaek NE, Berthelsen JG (1978) Carcinoma-in-situ of testis and orchiectomy. Lancet, 204–205
30. Skakkebaek NE (1979) Carcinoma-in-situ of testis in testicular feminization syndrome. Acta Pathol Microbiol Scand 87A:87–89
31. Krabbe S, Skakkebaek NE, Berthelsen JG (1979) High incidence of undetected neoplasia in maldescended testes. Lancet 999–1000
32. Anonymous (1980) Testicular biopsy for early detection of testicular tumors. Br Med J 426–427
33. Gehring GG et al. (1974) Malignant degeneration of

cryptorchid testes following orchiopexy. J Urol 112: 354

34. Wan SP, Uechi MD (1960) Seminoma in atrophic testis. Urology XVI:183–185
35. Carleton RL et al. (1953) Experimental teratomas of the testis. Cancer 6:464
36. Collins DH, Pugh RCB (1964) Classification and frequency of testicular tumors. Br J Urol 36:1
37. Batata M et al. (1980) Cryptorchidism and testicular cancer. J Urol 124:382
38. Whitaker RH (1970) Management of the undescended testis. Br J Hosp Med
39. Martin DC (1981) Malignancy and the undescended testis. In: Fonkalsrud EW, Mengel W (eds) The undes-

cended testis. Yearbook Med Publ, Chicago London, pp 144–156
40. Sedransk N, Cromie WJ (to be published) A Bayesian approach to joint incidence of rare medical conditions. J Am Stat Assoc
41. Myers MH, Hankey BF (1980) Cancer patient survival experience. Natl Inst Health Pub 80–2148:7–15
42. Skinner DG, Smith RB (1980) Treatment of testicular carcinoma. In: Haskell M, Parker R, Kline M (eds) Clinical oncology. Saunders, Philadelphia, pp 405–407
43. Knudson AG, Strong CC (1972) Mutation and cancer: a model for Wilms'tumor of the kidney. J Natl Cancer Inst 48:313

8 Examinations and Clinical Findings in Cryptorchid Boys

F. Hadžiselimović

8.1 Incidence

Cryptorchidism is the most frequent disorder of an endocrine gland. From the data available in various publications, premature males have an incidence of 9.22% while full-term boys have cryptorchidism in 5.83% of cases [1]. After 1 year, out of 88,526 patients only 1.82% had undescended testes [1]. The percentage remained the same until puberty [1]. Scorer and Farrington, however, found 30% cryptorchidism in premature babies and 3.4% in full-term newborns [2]. At the end of 12 months, 28 out of 3,612 babies still had cryptorchidism, an incidence of 0.8% [2]. These findings underline that, after the 1st year, spontaneous descent is unlikely to occur.

8.2 Position and Side Affected

With regard to the position of the undescended gonad taken from the published data of 39,895 cryptorchid boys, 8.08% (1,177 out of 14,548) had abdominally located testes, 62.76% (9,130 out of 13,518) had testes in an inguinal position, 23.81% (713 out of 2,985) had prescrotally located testes, and 10.93% (313 out of 2,717) had ectopic testes, including superficial ectopic testes [1]. In 2.6% (159 out of 6,127) there was aplasia or anorchia [1]. From 22,015 cryptorchid boys, 6,647 (30.19%) had bilateral cryptorchidism and 15,368 (69.81%) had unilateral maldescended testis [1]. The left side was affected in 6,631 out of 15,368 boys (30.12%) and the right side in 8,737 boys (69.69%).

Terms used to describe the position of the testes are diverse. From the histological point of view and from the point of subsequent fertility the following classification can be recommended:

1. Retractile testis
2. True cryptorchid testis
   a) Abdominally located
   b) Inguinally located
   c) Suprascrotally located
   d) Gliding
3. Ectopic testis

The retractile testis (German: *Pendelhoden*) is caused by an hyperactive cremaster muscle and has normal histology and fertility. With the patient in the cross-legged position the testis can be manipulated easily into the scrotum and it remains there for a while. About 50% of the children examined in our policlinic suspected of having maldescended testis displayed this characteristic.

The gliding testis can be manipulated into the scrotum, but after release it immediately returns to the position at the superficial inguinal pouch. These testes should be treated hormonally.

Testes located at the superficial inguinal pouch have often been described as ectopic (23%) due to a transverse obstructing fascia usually lying in the neck of the scrotum [2]. Our intraoperatively performed study on 66 cryptorchid boys showed that only two (3%) had a mechanical barrier on the way into the scrotum. Histological findings showing that epifascial "ectopias" have an altered rather than normal S/T count, also support our findings (Chap. 4.2.1.2). Consequently, only the true ectopias should not receive hormonal therapy as the treatment of the first choice. It also means that the term "ectopia" should be given to the testis found outside the normal range of movement, i.e. in a femoral, perineal, penile or pubic position.

Table 1. Syndromes frequently associated with cryptorchidism [21, 22]. *S*, growth retardation; *M*, mental retardation

Syndrome	S	M
Aarskog	+	(+)
Carpenter		+
Cleft lip palate, tetraphocomelia	+	+
Cryptophthalmos		(+)
Dubowitz		+
Gorlin frontometaphyseal dysplasia		(+)
Laurence-Moon-Bardet-Biedl	(+)	(+)
Lowe	+	+
Leopard	+	(+)
Meckel-Gruber	+	+
Noonan	+	+
Opitz		+
Prader-Labhart-Willi	+	+
Roberts	+	+
Rubinstein-Taybi	+	+
Seckel	+	+
Smith-Lemli-Opitz	+	+
Triploidy	+	+
Trisomy 13	+	+
Trisomy 18	+	+
XXXXY	+	+
4p	+	+
13q	+	+
18q	+	+
Prune belly	−	−

Table 2. Cryptorchidism frequency in chromosomal anomalies [21]

Anomaly	Frequency	%
Trisomy D	28/30	93.4
Trisomy E	11/16	68.8
Trisomy 21		?
Cat-eye Syndrome[a]	−	−
Autosomal deletion syndromes		
Chromosome 4 short-arm deletion	4/7	57
Chromosome 5 short-arm deletion	8/20	40
Chromosome D long-arm deletion	4/6	66
D-ring chromosome	6/8	74
Chromosome 18 short-arm deletion	2/7	27
Chromosome 18 long-arm deletion	5/9	55
18-ring chromosome	2/4	50
Klinefelter 47,XXY	12/276	4.3
Klinefelter 48,XXXY	0/7	−
Klinefelter 49,XXXXY	11/17	65.7

[a] Although renal malformation occurs in 100% of cat-eye syndrome cases, cryptorchidism relatively seldom parallels it

8.3 Concomitant Findings

8.3.1 Mental and Somatic Retardation

A connection between mental and somatic development and occurrence of cryptorchidism is often encountered (Tables 1, 2).

Of children with various cerebral lesions, 44% had uni- or bilateral cryptorchidism [3]. In children with meningomyelocele, 23% (6/23) had maldescended testes [4]. When the bony defect was above L_2, the incidence was 50% [4]. While only 67% of all meningomyelocele children had hydrocephalus, it was present in all meningomyelocele children with cryptorchidism [4].

Several chromosomal anomalies and syndromes are frequently associated with undescended testes (Tables 1, 2). All syndromes and chromosomal anomalies listed beside having cryptorchidism, frequently have mental and somatic retardation. This suggests that the causative factor of cryptorchidism is not primarily a genetic failure but more likely to be an intrauterine disturbance of the CNS and involving the hypothalamo-pituitary-gonadal axis development. The observations on anencephalic fetuses (Chap. 5) and on patients with Noonan's syndrome, where there is a disturbance of the pituitary-gonadal system in 71.4% (5/7) of the patients studied, additionally support this hypothesis [5].

8.3.2 Heredity

The hereditary tendency of undescended testes is a well-known phenomenon [1]. From 2,633 patients with undescended testes, 139 had a history of familial involvement, thus indicating a hereditary tendency in cryptorchid patients of 5.28% [1]. The occurrence of cryptorchid testes could be confirmed in 1.5%–4.0% of the fathers and in 6.2% of the brothers of patients with true undescended testes [6]. Bilateral undescended testes are associated with a higher risk for siblings [6]. The family data studied support the contention that both uni- and bilateral cryptorchidism have a nosological identity [6]. The mothers of patients with cryptorchidism have shorter menses and a delay in menarche [6, 7]. Therefore the hypothesis was formulated that pituitary hypogonadism of the mothers may be a predetermining factor for undescended testes in their sons [6].

A significantly higher content of α-fetoprotein (AFP) was found in the placenta of true cryptorchid boys (2α = 0.01 Wilcoxon test). All the placenta examined belonged to newborns with a birth weight of over 2,800 g and a gestational age of between 38–40 weeks. The median values of cryptorchid boys ($n = 4$) were 7.4 µg/mg of placentar tissue while those with normal descent ($n = 16$) had a median AFP value of 2,35 µg/mg. The cryptorchid children were operated upon between the ages of 1 1/2–2 years and cryptorchidism was definitively proven by the subsequent biopsy.

Further research into this field will elucidate the importance of these initial observations towards the etiology of cryptorchidism.

8.3.3 Torsion of Testis

Torsion of the testis has a dual pathogenesis, depending on the anatomical anomaly present, namely, intravaginal torsion or extravaginal torsion [8]. In cryptorchidism, the anatomical peculiarities ("bell-clapper" or expressed areolar connections between the parietal tunica vaginalis and surrounding fascias) are the rule rather than the exception, so that torsion, both intravaginal and extravaginal, occurs more frequently [8].

8.3.4 Hernias, Renal Failure, and Genital Malformations

The coincidence of the open processus vaginalis in boys with maldescended testes was 49.2% (7,701 of 15,653) [1]. Kleinteich summarized the various findings and compared three randomized groups of boys with cryptorchidism and found an occurrence of renal anomalies in 17.4% (157 of 903) and anomalies of external genitalia in 8.17% (199 of 2,437) [1]. This high incidence of renal failure and anomalies of the external genitalia was confirmed in another study, in which 237 consecutive cases of undescended testes were examined [9]. Renal agenesis was more common in the presence of cryptorchid testes than in the general population [9]. Unilateral renal agenesis may be associated with ipsilateral agenesis of the vas deferens and the testis, but agenesis of the contralateral vas deferens and testis is also described [9]. As the

17.4% incidence of renal anomalies is relatively high and the ultrasound examination a good noninvasive technique, we suggest that all boys with cryptorchidism should have an ultrasound examination of the abdomen undertaken.

8.3.5 Psychic Alterations

It is an empty sac, uni- or bilateral which most often brings the patients and their parents to the pediatric urologist. If cryptorchidism is bilateral sterility and feminization ensue. Sterility plays an important psychological role; the patient becomes depressed about his procreative inability and may fear homosexual attack [10]. Among his peers he is teased unmercifully [10]. If one testicle has descended he can still have children, but his body image is impaired and he feels defective genitally [10]. Many of these boys have learning disabilities and suffer from depression [10]. They become loners with serious behavioral disturbances [10]. Prophylaxis is primarily the role of the pediatrician. He should be able to recognize the psychological difficulties, reassure both child and parents and commence any necessary treatment.

8.4 Examination Technique

The position of the testis is easily determined provided:
1. Room and examiner's hands are warm
2. The boy examined is given time to relax and the examiner is not in a hurry
3. A warm bath is given, if necessary, to help distinguish between retractile and true cryptorchid testes.

Newborn babies are easy to examine because of their weak cremaster reflex and only scanty subcutaneous fat. After 6 months of life the examination should be started with the patient in a cross-legged position, in which the cremaster reflex is generally absent. Once the patient is sitting comfortably in the cross-legged position, most retractile testes descend spontaneously without being manipulated by the examiner.

Another helpful approach, particularly in older boys, is application of pressure on the femoral artery in the groin. If the testis is retractile it should immediately descend and remain in the scrotum for a while (Fig. 1a and b). The gonad should be manipulated gently into the scrotum with the thumb and the forefinger. The use of measurement in diagnosing the cryptorchid state, as suggested by Scorer and Farrington [2], does not seem to be of significant help to clinicians. The most important thing is that the testis has to lie within the scrotum, and if this is not achieved the histological changes described for cryptorchid testes occur, measurement notwithstanding.

If the testis has not reached the adequate scrotal position, it will be smaller in size, and the higher the testis the smaller and softer it usually is (Fig. 1c). These testes have an increasing tendency to being gliding and the scrotum is less well developed on the affected side [2].

The management of these high scrotal testes presents the most difficult diagnostic problems. The majority do have normal histology, but in a small proportion considerable damage to the gonad develops with time. Therefore, a careful annual check-up of the development and position of these gonads is recommended. Should any doubt about growth and position arise, hormonal treatment should be started, particularly if the testis becomes a gliding one.

Detailed pregnancy and familial histories are obligatory. A twofold greater frequency of undescended testis has been found among infants whose mothers took oral contraceptives within the 1st month of pregnancy [11]. The 90% confidence interval for the prevalence ratio was 0.9 to 3.9 [11]. Whether this excess is explained by a sampling variability or not is unknown. Another study on the boys whose mothers used diethylstilbestrol to prevent miscarriage showed a slightly higher than expected incidence of undescended testes, epididymal cysts, and other genitourinary abnormalities [12]. This would support the hypothesis that estrogen derivates taken throughout gestation increase the frequency of male offspring with cryptorchidism. Sixty percent of male offspring from pregnant mice treated with diethylstilbestrol during gestation were sterile and had uni- or bilateral intra-abdominal testes [13].

Measurements of height in numerous groups of patients with various testicular pathology have established that the average values are – with the exception of the group with testicular hypoplasia – higher than in the control group of somatosexually adequately developed and fertile men [14]. The differences are statistically significant in examinees with bilateral disturbance of descensus, in unilateral cryptorchids with normal spermatogenesis, in hypogonadotrophic eunuchs, and in patients with a Klinefelter syndrome [14]. In the latter group, the difference in average height from that of the control group is the most pronounced [14]. In another study, involving a smaller group of 101 cryptorchids, all patients reached normal adult height [15]. The conclusion to be drawn is that the deviation from normal growth in individual patients appeared to be related neither to their earlier undescended testes nor to successful therapy, but rather to their genetic background [15]. This latter group studied, however, was not divided according to fertility rating. The pubertal rating has to be performed generally according to Tanner. Careful examination of scrotal anatomy and testicular form is advised. The anatomy of the penis should also be carefully examined to exclude abnormalities, i.e. male pseudohermaphroditism with chordee, hypospadias, epispadias, etc. The stretched length of the flaccid penis (SPL) offers the most convenient means of reference for penile size and for comparison between subjects [16]. This measurement has been shown to correlate closely with erected penile length in 150 boys between 3 and 16 years [16]. The SPL is determined by direct measurement of the organ from the root of the penis at its junction with the pubis to the tip of its body (Table 3) [16]. To establish testicular volume, testis length and short diameter have to be estimated or the testis should be measured with Prader's

Table 3. Length of the stretched penis during childhood [19, 20]

Age (years)	Mean length (cm)	Mean circumference (cm)
Newborn	3.5 ± 0.4	3.3 ± 0.3
1–9	4–6	3.6–4.6
10	6.2	4.5
11	6.5	4.7
12	7.1	5.0
13	8.7	5.7
14	9.7	6.8
15	11.8	7.6
16	12.5	7.9
17	13.2	8.4

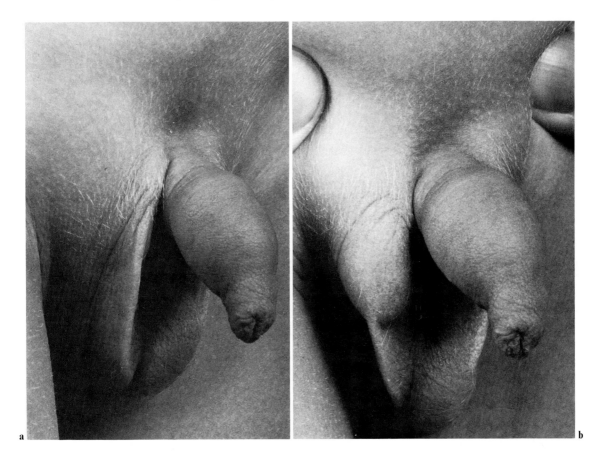

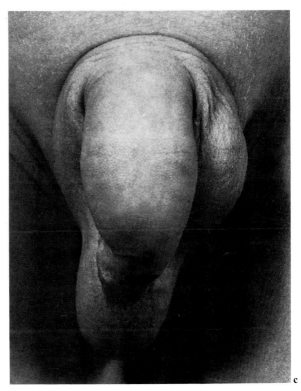

Fig. 1. a The right part of the scrotum is empty, indicating cryptorchidism. **b** Slight pressure applied on the femoral artery induces testicular descent. Only retractile testes descend with this maneuver. **c** The high scrotal testis, successfully treated with GnRH. The testis was previously located in the inguinal canal

Table 4. Testicular volume during childhood [17, 18]

Age (aears)	Mean long and short diameters [17] (mm)	Mean volume [18] (ml)
Newborn [17]	19 × 12	1.6 ± 0.4
1–9	15 × 10	≦ 1
10	18 × 11	1.2 ± 0.4
11	20 × 14	1.8 ± 0.8
12	23 × 18	4.0 ± 2.7
13	30 × 23	7.0 ± 4.5
14	34 × 25	10.8 ± 5.8
15	36 × 26	12.8 ± 5.4
16	38 × 27	14.4 ± 4.5
17	40 × 28	17.6 ± 4.0

orchidometer (Table 4). The epididymis has to be completely palpated to find various malformations such as a long-loop epididymis or partial agenesis of vas deferens. The looped epididymis could sometimes mimic atrophic testis and its descent could erroneously be interpreted as a descended atrophic testis when the testis is in fact located inguinally. Therefore, in all cases of atrophic testes within the scrotum, detailed palpation of the prescrotal and inguinal area with the patient lying down is mandatory. In cases where both testes are impalpable, ultrasound or even computer tomography is recommended. Endocrine parameters such as elevated levels of FSH, as well as failure of the plasma testosterone to rise after $3 \times 1,500$ IU HCG administered at 4-day intervals, have been used in an attempt to distinguish whether the testes are congenitally absent or remain abdominally located. If there is no testosterone rise and FSH basal levels are high it can be concluded that the testes are non-existant.

References

1. Kleinteich B, Hadžiselimović F, Hesse V, Schreiber G (1979) Kongenitale Hodendystopien. Georg Thieme, Leipzig
2. Scorer CG, Farrington HG (1971) Congenital deformities of the testis and epididymis. Butterworths London
3. Ankerhold J, Gressmann C (1979) Hodendescensusstörungen beim frühkindlichen Hirnschaden. Z Kinderheilkd 107:15–25
4. Kropp AK, Voeller KSK (1981) Cryptorchidism in meningomyelocele. J Pediatr 99:110–113
5. Okuyama A, Nishimoto N, Yoshioka T, Itatani H, Takaha M, Mizutani S, Aono T, Matsumoto K, Sonoda T (1981) Gonadal findings in cryptorchid boys with Noonan's phenotype. Eur Urol 7:274–277
6. Czeizel A, Erödi E, Joth J (1981) Genetics of undescended testis. J Urol 126:528–529
7. Schlack H, Schlack FH (1977) Maldescensus testis and maternal menarche. In: Bierich RJ, Roger K, Ranke BM (eds) Maldescensus testis. Urban & Schwarzenberg, München Wien Baltimore
8. Charny WC, Wolgin W (1957) Cryptorchidism. Hoeber-Harper Book, New York
9. Mercer S (1979) Agenesis or atrophy of the testis and vas deferens. Can J Surg 22:245–246
10. Bell IA (1974) Psychologic implications of scrotal sac and testes for the male child. Clin Pediatr 13:838–847
11. Rothman JK, Louik C (1978) Oral contraceptives and birth defects. N Engl J Med 299:522–524
12. Cosgrove MD, Bentun B, Henderson BE (1977) Male genitourinary abnormalities and maternal diethylstilbestrol. J Urol 117:220–222
13. McLachlan JA, Newbold RR, Bullock B (1975) Reproductive tract lesions in male mice exposed prenatally to diethylstilbestrol. Science 190:991–992
14. Raboch J Jr, Reisenauer R (1976) Analysis of body height in 829 patients with different forms of testicular pathology. Andrologia 8:265–268
15. Schnakenburg K von, Butenandt O, Knorr D (1977) Adult height of patients treated in childhood for undescended testes. Eur J Pediatr 126:85–87
16. Kogan JS (1981) Micropenis; etiologic and management considerations. In: Kogan JS, Hafez ESE (eds) Pediatric andrology. Martinus Nijhoff, The Hague, Boston London
17. Job JC, Pierson M (1981) Endocrinologie pédiatrique et croissance. Flammarion Médecine Sciences, Paris
18. Zachmann M, Prader A, Kind HP, Haefliger H, Buldinger H (1974) Testicular volume during adolescence. Cross-sectional and longitudinal studies. Helv Paediatr Acta 29:61–72
19. Schonefeld WA, Beebe GW (1942) Normal growth and variation in the male genitalia from birth to maturity. J Urol 48:759–777
20. Flatau E, Josefsberg F, Reisner SH, Bialik O, Laron Z (1975) Penile size in the newborn infant. J Pediatr 87:663
21. Egli F, Stalder G (1973) Malformations of kidney and urinary tract in common chromosomal aberrations. Humangenetik 18:1–15
22. Smith WD (1976) Recognizable patterns of human malformation. Saunders, Philadelphia London Toronto

9 Indications and Contraindications for Orchiopexy

F. Hinman, Jr.

The first treatment is often hormonal therapy with HCG, and more recently with GnRH, since waiting for spontaneous descent carries unacceptable hazards. Operative intervention is the second line of treatment, either by orchiopexy or, less often, by orchiectomy. Certain cases may best be managed by no treatment at all.

9.1 Perform Orchiopexy

Orchiopexy is usually resorted to when hormonal therapy fails after one or two trials. It may be the only effective therapy for the ectopic testis or one retained after previous hernioplasty. It is especially indicated in bilateral cases not responding to hormonal therapy. With the various technics described in Chap. 11, orchiopexy can effect scrotal placement of almost all cryptorchid testes. If it is performed early in life, some salvage of fertility can be expected.

However, if putting the testis in a normal position does not improve fertility or reduce the risk of malignancy, was the operation justified? Would removing the testis or even doing nothing further serve the child better? These alternatives to orchiopexy will be considered separately [4].

9.2 Perform Orchiectomy

If the testis is incapable of effective spermatogenesis, and since the cryptorchid testis has a greater chance of malignancy, orchiectomy may be the treatment of choice in certain cases. Such advice is not easy to give: the parent wants a whole child, and the surgeon is dedicated to correcting anatomical abnormalities.

Orchiectomy may be desirable treatment for unilateral abdominal testis and is indicated in the symptomatic testis after puberty.

Unilateral abdominal testes form a distinct subgroup in cryptorchidism, having rather specific characteristics which affect fertility and proneness to malignancy [3]. First, the testis often is less well developed, smaller in size with poorer germinal epithelium. Because improvement in fertility is not assured by orchiopexy for unilateral testes wherever situated [4], it will be less often expected for the testis in a high position. Secondly, associated abnormalities of the adnexae are more common [8, 9]. In one series, a quarter of all abdominal testes had agenesis of the epididymis or of a portion of the vas [5]. Thirdly, malignancy is more frequent in these testes. It is significant that about 50% of the tumors occur in high testes, even though the latter constitute only 15% of cryptorchid testes [1].

The testis symptomatic after puberty, if unilateral, may require treatment because it is susceptible to trauma. Orchiopexy is not indicated, since spermatogenesis cannot be restored. The risk of malignancy is less than the risk of operation, unless the testis is intra-abdominal, in which case removal may be warranted [6].

Bilateral orchiectomy for intra-abdominal testes may also be advisable for the young man showing declining serum testosterone levels with rising levels of LH (an indication of early Leydig cell failure): the purpose is to avoid the risk of later malignancy for a patient who in any case requires supplemental testosterone.

9.3 Omit Surgical Treatment

No further treatment may be indicated for boys with: (1) severe mental incompetency, (2) inability to ejaculate effectively, or (3) certain major genetic disorders.

Mental incompetency, evidenced by severe and profound retardation, may be defined as inability to obtain a Stanford-Binet test score of above 35, where 100 is considered normal. Boys with this degree of disability are wards of society. Should orchiopexy allow them to procreate, their children would also become society's responsibility. Their activities then must be restricted to avoid impregnation of others. Further, if they were to have a child, their independence will be further limited by the need for someone else to help them with its care. Thus, even though the parents desire these retarded boys to be made as normal as possible, the needs of society may be stronger.

Failure of ejaculation, with severe meningomyelocele and similar congenital neurologic disorders, makes restoration of sperm to the ducts by orchiopexy of no avail. In the developed triad (prune-belly) syndrome, the prostate is so deficient in substance and the prostatic urethra so dilated that impregnation is impossible.

Genetic defects producing major developmental deficiencies may be accompanied by failure of testicular descent. Azoospermia often follows chromosomal disturbances, especially Klinefelter's syndrome with XXY and XXXY karyotypes [7] (although fertility has been described in XXY–XY mosaics) [2, 10]. Aplasia of the germinal epithelium is characteristic of the Sertoli cell only syndrome. Inborn errors of testosterone biosynthesis or gonadal dysgenesis occur in some forms of male pseudohermaphroditism with resulting sterility. Orchiopexy will not correct these deficits, so that no treatment (or orchiectomy in certain cases) would be preferable.

The laudable goal of the surgeon to restore anatomical relationships to normal may need to be altered in some cases because of the unnecessary risks of malignancy and the inability to achieve fertility.

References

1. Campbell HE (1942) Incidence of malignant growth of the undescended testicle: A critical and statistical study. Arch Surg 44:353–369
2. Court-Brown WM, Mantle DJ, Buckton KE, Tough IM (1964) Fertility in an XY/XXY male married to a translocation heterozygote. J Med Genet 1:35–38
3. Hinman F Jr (1979) Unilateral abdominal cryptorchidism. J Urol 122:71–75
4. Hinman F Jr (1980) Alternatives to orchiopexy. J Urol 123:548–551
5. Marshall FF, Shermeta DW (1979) Epididymal abnormalities associated with undescended testis. J Urol 121:341–343
6. Martin DC, Menck HR (1975) Undescended testis: Management after puberty. J Urol 114:77–79
7. Paulsen CA (1974) The testes. In: Williams RH (ed) Textbook of endocrinology. Saunders, Philadelphia, p 323
8. Scorer CG, Farrington GH (1971) Congenital deformities of the testis and epididymis. Appleton-Century-Crofts, New York
9. Scorer CG, Farrington GH (1981) Congenital anomalies of the testis: Cryptorchidism, testicular torsion, and inguinal hernia and hydrocele. In: Harrison JH (ed) Urology, 4th eds. Saunders, Philadelphia, p 10
10. Warburg E (1963) A fertile patient with Klinefelter's syndrome. Acta Endocrinol (Copenh) 43:12–26

10 Hormonal Treatment

F. Hadžiselimović

10.1 HCG Treatment

The ultimate aim of all therapeutic approaches to cryptorchidism is to achieve intrascrotally located testes. This can be effected either by surgical or by hormonal treatment. Although surgical treatment was inaugurated in 1820 by Rosenmerkel [1] and hormonal treatment about 100 years later [2], the latter is today the treatment of first choice.

Until recently HCG was the only mode of treatment. In the past 15 years different schedules have been proposed, each differing in the amount of HCG to be given and the duration of the treatment. The doses varied considerably, ranging between 3,000 and 50,000 IU/treatment [1]; duration varied from 3 days to 1 year [3]. The results of hormonal treatment varied considerably, from nil or very poor [4, 5] to 70% and 100% [6, 7].

Such variations can be explained by a different population of patients in pediatric versus urological practices. Particularly pediatric urologists had a preselected group of patients, those in whom conservative treatment failed.

The largest series of HCG-treated boys was reported by Bergada in 1979 [9]. He treated 1,204 patients and had success in 40% of the bilateral and 30% of the unilateral cryptorchid boys. This success rate is lower than that of Bierich (338/612 patients; 55%) [10], Knorr (300/574 patients; 52%) [11], and Pagliano-Sassi (115/213 patients; 54%) [12]. The explanation for these differences is probably the inclusion of gliding testes, which have been treated in the three latter groups but not by Bergada [9].

However, because of the painful mode of application, psychic alterations and effect on the growth of the genitalia, this treatment is no longer recommended as the therapy of first choice.

10.2 GnRH Treatment

The role and the physiological importance of GnRH have been studied extensively during the past 10 years. GnRH is produced by *Eminentia mediana* and acts as a "chemotransmitter." Through the pituitary-portal system it is delivered to the gonadotropin-producing cells within the pituitary. GnRH was detected by an immunohistochemical method in the corpus amygdaloideum, nucleus habenulae, and formatio reticularis [13]. Cathecholamine stimulates the secretion of GnRH but also an involvement of dopamine, serotonin, acetylcholine, melatonin, histamine, and GABA have been studied [14]. GnRH stimulates the pituitary to release LH and FSH. After the GnRH is bound to the cell wall receptors, the activation of cAMP results and an influx of Ca^{++} in the cell occurs [15]. This activation of cAMP induces a further activation of protein kinase and phosphorylase reaction at secretory granules, ribosomes, and chromatin of the nucleus, and enables a Ca^{++} reflux from mitochondria [15]. Ca^{++} is a modulator of enzymatic processes and has an inhibitory action on cAMP ("intracellular negative feedback") [15, 16]. Emiocytosis occurs within minutes via activation of the contractile microtubular system [15]. Several hours are necessary for the hypotrophy of the Golgi apparatus to develop [16]. There is still discussion on whether there are two different cell types for LH and FSH or if the single cell type secretes both hormones.

The first attempt to treat cryptorchid boys with GnRH was made in 1972 by Bergada et al. [17] and proved to be unsuccessful. The first favorable results were observed by Bartsch and Frick, who used intramuscular injections of GnRH [18]. They were able to achieve success in 84% of their cases. In 1974, Dahlén et al. [19] proved that an intranasal application of GnRH stimulates the pituitary to release LH

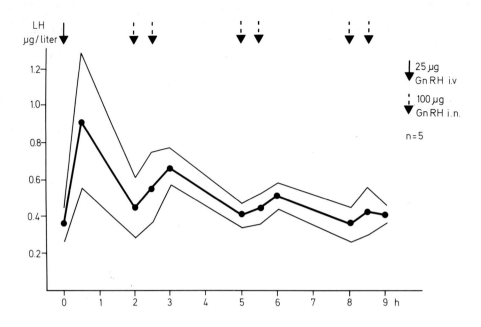

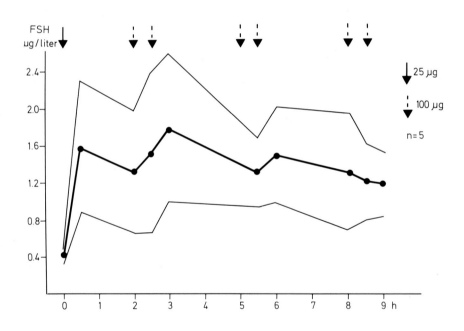

Fig. 1. Gonadotropin profile after repeated GnRH stimulation (6 × 100 μg intranasally). (With permission from B. Westphal [16])

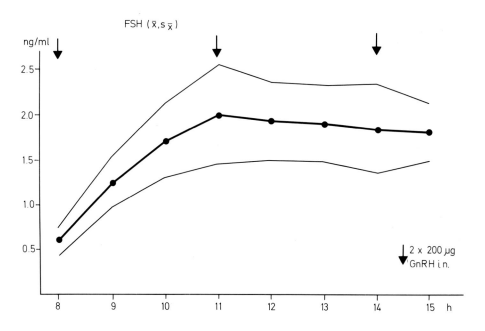

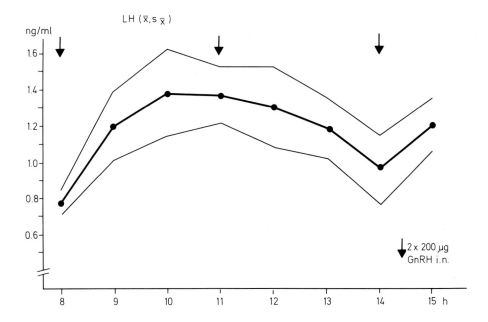

Fig. 2. Profile of gonadotropin secretion after administration of 400 µg GnRH thrice. (With permission from B. Hoecht [16])

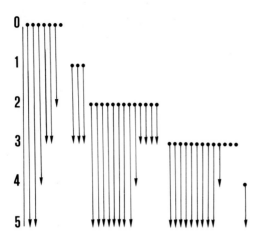

Fig. 3. Success rate and position of testes before and after GnRH treatment. For explanation of the position see Table 1

and FSH. The 200 µg nasal application is equivalent to a 2–10 µg i.v. application [16]. The lowest dose of GnRH necessary to stimulate LH significantly is 3 µg i.v. and of FSH about 25 µg [20]. Maximum plasma values were achieved 30–45 min after stimulation [16].

Repeated GnRH stimulation (6 × 100 µg intranasally) leads to a downregulation of the pituitary receptors (Fig. 1a, b). This does not occur when the periods between stimulations are prolonged (Fig. 2a, b).

Pharmacokinetic and metabolic studies of GnRH showed that this peptide is metabolized and eliminated quickly in humans and animals [16]. Secretion of gonadotropin, due to receptor stimulation, was maintained for several hours, while the serum plasma peptide level quickly diminished. In vivo, the inactivation of GnRH occurs quickly. It is metabolized to oligopeptides which are biologically ineffective [16]. These oligopeptides are excreted in urine. The intact peptide structure of GnRH is mandatory for its biological activity [16]. The main metabolites of GnRH are: (2–10)-nonapeptide, (3–10)-octapeptide, (1–6)-hexapeptide, and (7–10)-tetrapeptide [16]. In vitro, metabolism into (1–5)-pentapeptide and (6–10)-pentapeptide was also observed. The highest amount of GnRH is metabolized in the liver and the kidneys [16].

Pirazzoli et al. [21] treated cryptorchid boys with two different schedules: group A was treated with 6 × 100 µg nasal spray daily in each nostril (total 1,200 µg/day), while group B received 2 × 500 µg/day (total 1,000 µg) for a treatment period of 7 days.

Out of 47 patients treated, 14 (29.8%) showed a positive response with descent of the testis into the scrotum. Of these, 5 (21.7%) belonged to group A and 9 (37.5%) to group B. Sixteen children showed a partial response; of these 9 (39.1%) belonged to group A and 7 (29.2%) to group B. This study showed that nonpulsatile GnRH application in prepubertal cryptorchid boys also induces testicular descent. Basal LH and FSH plasma values remained the same before and after treatment. The pituitary response of LH (area under the curve) was significantly higher in the children who responded to therapy. A positive correlation was found between response to therapy and pituitary reserve (peak and area of the curve) of LH before treatment ($P < 0.05$). Thirty-three boys were treated with HCG after GnRH therapy: three (9%) from the group who partially responded to GnRH therapy had a total descent of the testes after HCG.

Happ and co-workers treated 25 patients aged 1–11 years suffering from uni- or bilateral cryptorchidism with GnRH nasal spray [22, 23]. All patients showed P_1-stage pubertal development. Sixteen patients also had 17-ketosteroids and 18 had PBI, T3, and T4 plasma values within the normal range. Estimation of stimulation values after bolus GnRH application showed that the peak values for LH in cryptorchid boys were significantly lower than those in boys with normally descended testes.

The position of the testes was determined independently by at least two qualified doctors. The checks were performed weekly. If one of the pathological testicular positions (0–3, Table 1) was transformed into a physiological position this was considered as a success. If descent, for example, from the abdominal into the inguinal position was noted at the end of the treatment, this was considered as partial success [22, 23].

Twenty-five patients received 6 × 200 µg GnRH nasal spray/day for a maximum of 10 weeks. The testes descended in the majority of treated patients in the period from 2 to 5 weeks after treatment commenced (Fig. 3). Six months after therapy cessation, 12% (3/25) had suffered a relapse. No side effects, particularly no psychic changes or changes in the

Table 1. Nomenclature of the position of the testes in the study of Happ et al. [22, 23]

Class	Position
0	Intra-abdominal or absent
1	Inguinal (fixed)
2	Inguinal (movable)
3	Inguinally located: it is possible to move the testis into the scrotum, but it returns to its former position immediately after being released (gliding)
4	High scrotal (*Pendelhoden*)
5	Scrotal (permanent)

growth and appearance of the genitalia, were detected. Also, no antibodies against GnRH were determined at the end of treatment.

A controlled *double-blind study* was carried out as a multicenter study in Zürich, Frankfurt, Graz, and Vienna [24, 25]. Only healthy prepubertal boys who were $1^1/_2$–12 years old with uni- or bilateral cryptorchidism participated. None of the boys had ever been treated for cryptorchidism before. Boys with retractile testes or with testes which could be manipulated into the scrotum or which had been observed in the scrotum were not included. Parents consented to the trial and the patients were randomly and blindly allocated to GnRH or placebo therapy. GnRH 100 μg was sprayed 6 times daily into each nostril (total dose 1.2 mg) [24, 25].

Included in this study were 28 boys with bilateral and 56 boys with unilateral cryptorchidism. Forty-six boys with a total of 61 undescended testes received GnRH spray, while 38 boys with a total of 51 undescended testes received a placebo.

There was complete descent of 23 testes in boys treated with GnRH and one testis in a boy treated with a placebo. The position of 17 GnRH-treated and seven placebo-treated testes improved. The position of 12 GnRH-treated and 29 placebo-treated testes was unchanged. Nine testes treated with GnRH and 14 treated with placebo were never palpated. There was no statistical correlation between age and response to nasal GnRH. The lowest success rate was seen in the department of urology. None of the patients had developed antibodies to GnRH. The treatment was well tolerated and no side effects, particularly no growth of testes or penis, were observed. The improved position

found in a few boys treated with a placebo (and possibly also that in some boys treated with GnRH) can probably be explained by the fact that most children are more relaxed after repeated examinations [24].

Areas under the curves of GnRH-stimulated LH-release patterns before and after therapy were found statistically undistinguishable by the three groups participating in the study. Among the patients in the Frankfurt group, a statistical increase in GnRH stimulated LH-release was found after therapy ($P < 0.05$). No significant changes were found in any placebo group. GnRH-treated groups in three of the laboratories responded to i.v. GnRH application with a significant decrease of FSH release after therapy cessation ($P < 0.05$ to $P < 0.01$ – Wilcoxon test). Again, no significant changes were observed during the placebo treatment [25].

Intranasal application of GnRH did not alter basal testosterone serum levels in the subjects examined in the three laboratories, although a significant increase of testosterone serum levels ($P < 0.05$) was found in boys treated in the Zürich center [25]. No significant differences in hormone levels could be detected in boys who had not responded to treatment or in those in whom a descent, either partial or complete, occurred [25].

In general, the main objection to hormonal treatment is that only a retractile testis responds to the treatment, not a true cryptorchid testis. Bearing in mind that in retractile testes fertility in adulthood is normal, we performed a *randomized study* on 60 cryptorchid patients. The position of the gonad was verified by two pediatric surgeons and all boys had both chronological and bone age determined. According to the protocol, the children were randomly selected to be either immediately operated upon or treated with GnRH. No treated children had had previous treatment with HCG [26]. The randomized groups operated upon were compared histologically according to the quality of their testicular tissue. To complete this study, a third group (boys unsuccessfully treated with HCG) was also examined histologically. Of the cryptorchid boys, 56% (17/30) were successfully treated with GnRH while 34% (13/30) did not respond positively [26, 27]. The majority of the cryptorchid testes (78%; 37/47) were located in the inguinal canal before treatment

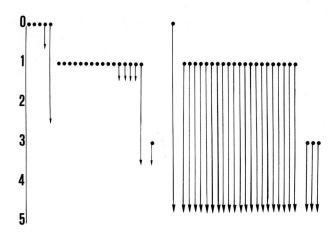

Fig. 4. Success rate and position of the testes in randomized study; before and after treatment with GnRH. *0*, abdominal or absent; *1*, inguinal (unmovable); *2*, inguinal (movable); *3*, at annulus inguinalis superficialis; *4*, high scrotal; *5*, scrotal

(Fig. 4). All testicular biopsies revealed histological changes typical of a cryptorchid gonad (reduced number of spermatogonia, thickening of peritubular connective tissue, atrophy of Leydig cells), indicating that only true cryptorchid boys were treated. The GnRH-treated group had an S/T count of 0.38 ± 0.52 and a tubule diameter of 51 μ $\pm$ 7 μ. The HCG-treated group had an S/T count of 0.35 ± 0.57 and a tubule diameter of 50 μ $\pm$ 4 μ, while the surgically treated group had an S/T count of 0.43 ± 0.7 and a tubule diameter of 50 μ $\pm$ 3 μ. With this treatment neither further diminution nor improvement of germ-cell count was achieved (Tables 2–4).

There was no correlation between the number of spermatogonia and a thickening and collagenization of the peritubular connective tissue. However, in those boys in whom the Leydig cells appeared more frequently within the interstitium, the peritubular connective tissue was least altered. The morphology of the Leydig cells was evidently changed after GnRH treatment. Three different types of Leydig cells were encountered:

1. Precursor Leydig cells, differentiating from the peritubular fibroblasts (Fig. 5)
2. A transient form (Fig. 6)
3. Juvenile Leydig cells (Fig. 7)

Table 2. Chronological and bone age, spermatogonia count, and tubule diameter after unsuccessful treatment with GnRH only

Pt.	Age (years)	Bone age (years)	S/T count	Tubule diameter (μ)
1	2.00	1.50	0.02	66
2	1.58	1.75	1.64	65
3	5.91	4.00	0.24	57
4	2.41	1.50	0.00	49
5	3.16	4.00	0.40	55
6	4.41	3.00	0.01	50
7	2.16	2.00	0.26	48
8	2.50	2.50	0.08	49
9	2.08	1.00	0.16	54
10	2.66	1.50	0.12	40
11	2.00	2.00	0.78	52
12	5.08	2.50	0.00	44
13	2.00	2.00	1.30	52
Mean	2.91	2.25	0.38	51
$\pm$ SD	1.35	0.93	0.52	7

Table 3. Chronological and bone age, spermatogonia count, and tubule diameter without hormonal treatment

Pt.	Age (years)	Bone age (years)	S/T count	Tubule diameter (μ)
1	4.66	4.00	0.00	54
2	5.90	5.50	0.01	51
3	2.00	2.00	1.46	53
4	2.08	2.00	0.04	53
5	2.16	2.00	0.04	45
6	3.00	3.00	0.04	52
7	1.33	1.00	0.10	49
8	3.33	3.00	0.66	43
9	5.75	5.50	1.94	52
10	3.58	3.00	0.02	47
Mean	3.37	3.1	0.43	50
$\pm$ SD	1.60	1.50	0.70	3

Table 4. Chronological and bone age, spermatogonia count, and tubule diameter after unsuccessful HCG treatment

Pt.	Age (years)	Bone age (years)	S/T count	Tubule diameter (μ)
1	1.25	1.50	2.10	51
2	3.33	2.50	0.08	51
3	2.91	3.00	0.00	45
4	4.91	5.00	0.01	46
5	4.41	5.00	0.69	48
6	0.66	0.75	0.01	60
7	5.75	5.00	0.58	57
8	5.75	3.50	0.00	48
9	6.50	2.50	0.36	51
10	5.50	5.50	0.40	50
11	2.00	2.00	0.00	52
12	2.66	2.50	0.00	43
13	1.50	1.50	0.72	57
14	1.91	2.50	0.02	50
Mean	3.50	2.95	0.35	50
±SD	1.94	1.51	0.57	4

Table 5. Basal gonadotropin values in three groups of cryptorchid boys

Group		Gonado-tropin	Before treatment (IU/litre)	After treatment (IU/litre)
Success	I	LH	2	3.8
No success	II	LH	1.7	2.6
Surgery	III	LH	1.7	
Success	I	FSH	0.8	0.8
No success	II	FSH	0.92	0.88
Surgery	III	FSH	1.08	

Table 6. Peak (30 min) gonadotropin values in three groups of cryptorchid boys studied

Group		Gonado-tropin	Before treatment (IU/litre)	After treatment (IU/litre)
Success	I	LH	6.8	9.6
No success	II	LH	8.8	4.8[a]
Surgery	III	LH	6.6	
Success	I	FSH	3.05	2.0
No success	II	FSH	3.0	1.16[b]
Surgery	III	FSH	3.4	

[a] $2\alpha = 0.01$ (median values: Wilcoxon rank sum test for unpaired data was performed), compared to I, II, III before treatment
[b] Only compared to III, $2\alpha = 0.01$

A typical feature of GnRH treatment was the marked mobilization of precursor Leydig cells. There were no adult Leydig cells with crystalloids of Reinecke within the interstitium. The juvenile Leydig cells had an increased amount of lipoid droplets in their cytoplasm (Fig. 7).

The changes within the Sertoli cells, particularly after GnRH treatment, were always present (Fig. 8). Their cytoplasm was rich with lipoid droplets and invaginations appeared at the nucleus (Fig. 8). A peripherally located nucleolus was prominent.

In our randomized study, nor changes in the basal LH and FSH before or after treatment occurred (Table 5) [28]. The 30 min stimulation plasma values for LH were significantly lower in the unsuccessfully treated group immediately after treatment was terminated (Table 6) [28]. The 30 min stimulation FSH values showed no significant decreasing tendency (Table 6). The estimation of first-morning-void urine (FMV) correlates to the gonadotropin values of 24 h urine [29]. Thus the FMV can be used as a parameter of daily gonadotropin secretion [29]. In our groups no difference before or after treatment was found (Table 7). The conclusion to be drawn is that after 4 weeks of therapy, with 1.2 mg GnRH daily, no enlargement of the gonadotropin stores within the pituitary and no influence upon basal gonadotropin se-

Table 7. FMV urine before and after GnRH treatment

	LH		FSH	
	n	(U/g creatinine)	n	(U/g creatinine)
Before successful GnRH treatment	7	2.9±1.9	7	3.3±4.2
After successful GnRH treatment	8	3.3±1.8	8	2.6±3.3
Before unsuccessful GnRH treatment	6	3.1±1.8	6	2.6±1.5
After unsuccessful GnRH treatment	8	3.1±1.6	8	2.2±1.6
Without GnRH treatment (surgery only)	11	2.2±1.5	11	2.3±1.6
Normal population control group	35	2.5±0.6	35	2.5±0.4

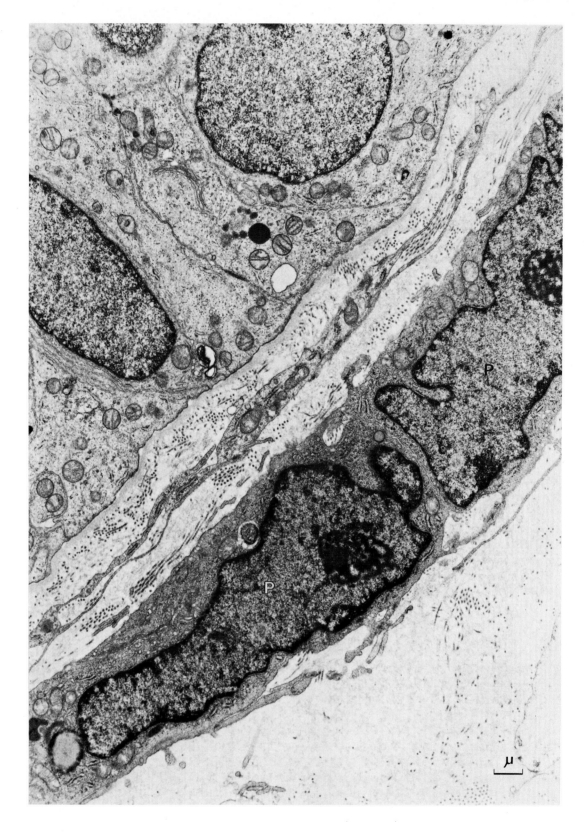

Fig. 5. Precursor Leydig cells (*P*)

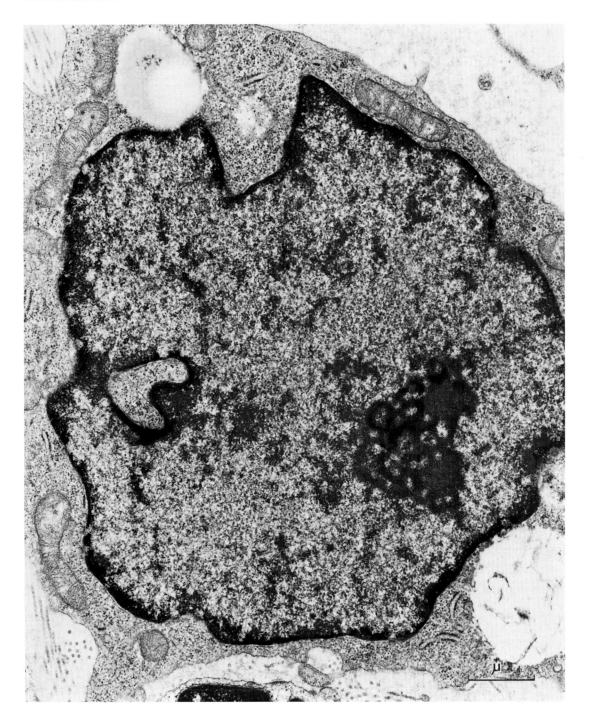

Fig. 6. Transitional stage of Leydig cell

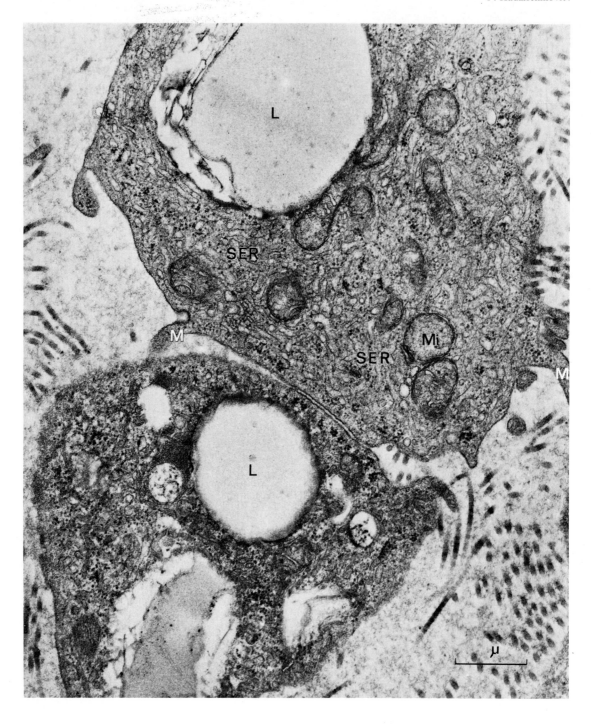

Fig. 7. Cytoplasm of the juvenile Leydig cells. Under GnRH stimulation the amount of smooth endoplasmic reticulum (*SER*) increases. *L*, lipoid droplets; *M*, microvilli; *Mi*, mitochondria

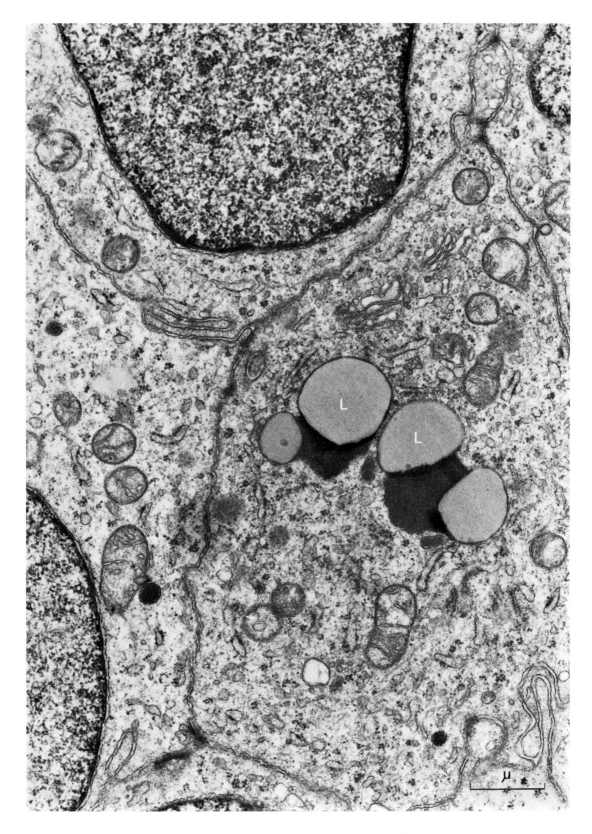

Fig. 8. Cytoplasm of the Sertoli cells after GnRH treatment. There is an increase in lipoid droplets (*L*) and cell organelles

cretion was achieved. Furthermore, FMV data is identical to the data obtained from the control group of prepubertal boys, although the standard deviation in the cryptorchid group is higher (Table 7). The latter further suggests that there exists a heterogeneity among boys with cryptorchidism.

To find whether additional HCG treatment after unsuccessful GnRH treatment increases the success rate, a further clinical study was attempted. Sixty patients aged between 10 months and 14 years were treated with GnRH-decapeptide nasal solution. Out of 37 who were outpatients in our polyclinic, 26 had unilateral and 11 had bilateral cryptorchid testes. The remaining boys (13 unilateral, 10 bilateral) received treatment from their own pediatricians. The position of the testes prior to treatment in our polyclinic was abdominal (8.3%), inguinal (54.2%), and superscrotal (37.5%). The duration of therapy was 4 weeks (Fig. 9). In this period, *200 μg of GnRH was sprayed thrice daily in each nostril* (total 1.2 mg/day). All the boys were subjected to a weekly check-up to assess the position of the gonads and the patient's general health. Partial descent was defined as a change from the previous position into the lower inguinal or superscrotal location. The patients with partial descent together with those with gliding testes were subsequently treated with HCG. In 37 patients the position of the testes was checked 6 months after completion of therapy. In all the operated patients (n = 7), the position of the gonad and the morphology of the epididymis and testes were determined.

A success rate of 79.5% was achieved in unilateral cryptorchid boys. Using only GnRH, success rates of 57.7% and 61.5% were realized in our polyclinic and by the pediatricians respectively. Subsequent HCG treatment resulted in a 26.9% additional success rate in our poly-

clinic and 7.7% by practitioners. A success rate of 81% was achieved in bilateral cryptorchid boys. Utilizing only GnRH, success rates of 63.6% and 65% were achieved in our polyclinic and by the pediatricians respectively. Additional HCG treatment resulted in a 22.7% additional success rate in our polyclinic and 10% by practitioners (Tables 8, 9). Six months later, six testes had suffered a relapse (14.5%). Thus from our polyclinic-treated patients, 73% of the testes remained descended 6 months after the cessation of therapy. Two years after treatment, additionally three more testes (7.3%) had suffered relapses. Thus, after 2 years, 67% of successfully treated testes remained descended.

In five out of seven patients the following morphological abnormalities were found at surgery: long-loop epididymis (n = 1), complete dissociation of epididymis and testis (n = 2), intravaginal canalicular testis (n = 1), and a large open processus vaginalis with short funiculus spermaticus (n = 1).

The mean S/T count was 0.22 ± 0.29. In boys in whom the treatment was not successful, the S/T count remained unchanged compared with those treated unsuccessfully with only GnRH or surgical methods. Electron-microscopic findings confirmed that the Leydig cells were stimulated. Mainly fetal and A_p spermatogonia were observed. There were no A_d and B spermatogonia or spermatocytes of the first order in the seminiferous tubule.

The lack of descent together with an impaired 30 min LH response to GnRH at the end of the treatment (6 × daily) [28] could be explained by a receptor downregulation of pituitary LH cells after prolonged GnRH treatment. Alternatively, a more severely impaired LH reserve in these cryptorchid boys could be exhausted by GnRH treatment administered six times daily leading to diminished LH secretion which cannot induce descent. Downregulation

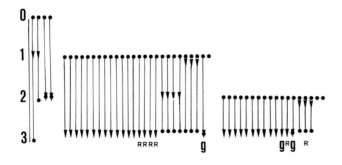

Fig. 9. Success rate and position of cryptorchid testes before and after treatment. The position at the end of GnRH treatment is indicated by the *arrow*, while the final position after additional HCG application is shown with the *point* (●). (*R*), relapse; *G*, the gliding testes were additionally treated with HCG; *0*, abdominal; *1*, inguinal; *2*, suprascrotal; *3*, scrotal

may not occur when GnRH is applied only three times daily [16].

The dosage and schedule of the subsequent HCG treatment, in unsuccessfully treated boys with GnRH, is based on the studies of testosterone dynamics after HCG injections by Forest et al. [30, 31]. The HCG concentrations, measured 4 days after injection, were shown to be several times higher than any physiological LH concentration [30, 31]. Furthermore, maximum testosterone levels were observed 72–120 h after HCG. A supposed optimum HCG dose of 50–100 U/kg body weight injected at intervals of at least 5 days formed the basis of the practical scheme of three injections over 3 weeks [30, 31].

A possible explanation for the better results achieved with a combination of GnRH followed by HCG is that GnRH releases LH and also an appropriate amount of FSH. The FSH increase mobilizes more LH receptors, probably by recruitment of Leydig cells from fibroblasts [28]. This induces a synthesis of androgen-binding protein (ABP), thus resulting in a higher local testosterone concentration than could be achieved with HCG treatment alone. A stimulation of recruited juvenile Leydig cells with additional HCG promotes the full development of these cells and produces a higher local testosterone concentration. This local increase in testosterone is responsible for the differentiation and further development of the epididymis and ultimately for descent [28]

The relapse by 14.5% of the patients within 6 months of completion of hormone treatment is comparable to that described in the literature [10]. With few exceptions, all the patients who experienced a relapse between 6 months and 2 years reacted positively to a repetition of GnRH treatment. This indicates that a relapse encountered after a long period should be hormonally retreated.

It is important to stress that in boys who were treated unsuccessfully in whom a testicular biopsy could be obtained, no inhibition or stimulation of the germ cells by this combined ther-

apy could be seen. Clinically, a slight penile enlargement has been observed following the HCG application in combined treatment.

Out of 171 GnRH-treated cryptorchid children published in the literature, three experienced discomfort in the inguinal region, five tended to be aggressive, and two had occasional penile erections. One case of penile growth and one case of testicular growth were also observed. No other adverse side effects were seen, nor were antibodies against GnRH detected [16].

Table 8. Success rate of combined therapy in 39 unilateral cryptorchid boys

	GnRH	GnRH +HCG	Success	No success
Our polyclinic	15/26 (57.7%)	7/26 (26.9%)	22/26 (84.6%)	4/26 (15.4%)
Pediatricians	8/13 (61.5%)	1/13 (7.7%)	9/13 (69.2%)	4/13 (30.8%)
Total	23/39 (59%)	8/39 (20%)	31/39 (79.5%)	8/39 (20.5%)

Table 9. The rate of successfully descended testes after hormonal treatment in 42 bilateral cryptorchid testes

	GnRH	GnRH +HCG	Success	No success
Our polyclinic	14/22 (63.6%)	5/22 (22.7%)	19/22 (86.3%)	3/22 (13.7%)
Pediatricians	13/20 (65.0%)	2/20 (10.0%)	15/20 (75.0%)	5/20 (25.0%)
Total	27/42 (64%)	7/42 (17.4%)	34/42 (81.0%)	8/42 (19.0%)

References

1. Rosenmerkel JF (1820) Über die Radikalkur des in der Weiche liegenden Testikels. Lindauer Verlag, München
2. Schapiro B (1931) Ist der Kryptorchismus chirurgisch oder hormonell zu behandeln? Dtsch Med Wochenschr 57:718
3. Kleinteich B, Hadžiselimović F, Hesse V, Schreiber G (1979) Kongenitale Hodendystopien. VEB, Georg Thieme, Leipzig
4. Deming C (1952) The evaluation of hormonal therapy in cryptorchidism. J Urol 68:354–357
5. Lawrence CH, Harrison AM (1937) Use of the gonadotropic hormone of pregnancy urine in the treatment of male sexual underdevelopment. N Engl J Med 217:89–94
6. Cernea R (1951) Zur Hormonbehandlung des Kryptorchismus. Hippocrates 22:241
7. Beatgen D (1970) Behandlungsergebnisse des Testis mobilis und der ein- und beidseitigen Retentio testis inguinalis mit Primogonyl. Med Welt I:313–315
8. Kunstadter RH (1941) The hormone treatment of cryptorchidism: Eight years' experience. Urol Cutaneous Rev 45:81–85
9. Bergada C (1979) Clinical treatment of cryptorchidism. In: Bierich JR, Giarola A (eds) Cryptorchidism. Academic Press, London
10. Bierich JR (1981) Gonadotropin therapy for the undescended testis. In: Kogan JS, Hafez ESE (eds) Pediatric andrology. Martinus Nijhoff, The Hague, Boston London
11. Knorr D (1970) Diagnose und Therapie der Descensusstörungen des Hodens. Pädiatr Praxis 9:299–304
12. Pagliano-Sassi L (1979) Significance and results of medical treatment in cryptorchidism. In: Bierich JR, Giarola A (eds) Cryptorchidism. Academic Press, London
13. Barry J (1976) Immunohistochemical localization of hypothalamic hormones (especially LRF) at the light microscopy level. In: Labrie F, Mestes J, Pelletier G (eds) Hypothalamus and endocrine functions. Plenum Press, New York
14. Krieger DT (1976) Neuroendocrinology. In: The year in endocrinology 1975–1976. Plenum Press, New York
15. Lacy PE (1967) The pancreatic beta-cell. Structure and functions. N Engl J Med 276:187–195
16. Ohe, M von der: Wissenschaftliche Monographie, Kryptocur, Höchst, Frankfurt a.M. 1982
17. Bergada C, Mancini RE, Vilar O, Rivarola MA, Calamera JC, Bianculli C, Schally AW, Kastin AJ (1972) Effect of chronic administration of synthetic LH-RH-FSH-RH on prepubertal boys and in hypogonadotropic hypogonadism. Serono Research Foundation, Proceedings of the conference held at Acapulco, Mexico, June 28–July 1, 1972
18. Bartsch G, Frick J (1974) Therapeutic effects of luteinizing hormone-releasing hormone (LH-RH) in cryptorchidism. Andrologia 6:197–201
19. Dahlén HG, Keller E, Schneider HPG (1974) Linear dose dependent LH release following intranasally sprayed LH. Horm Metab Res 6:510–513
20. Gonzales Barcena D, Kastin AJ, Schalch DS, Bermudez JA, Lee D, Arimura A, Ruelas J, Zepeda I, Schally AV (1973) Synthetic LH-releasing hormone (LH-RH) administered to normal men by different routes. J Clin Endocr Metab 37:481
21. Pirazzoli P, Zappulla F, Bernardi F, Villa MP, Aleksandrowicz A, Scandola A, Stancari P, Cicognani A, Cacciari E (1978) Luteinising hormone-releasing hormone nasal spray as therapy for undescended testicle. Arch Dis Child 53:235–238
22. Happ J, Kallmann F, Krawehl C, Neubauer M, Beyer J (1975) Intranasal GnRH therapy of maldescended testes. Horm Metab Res 7:440
23. Happ J, Kallmann F, Krawehl C, Neubauer M, Krause U, Demisch K, Sandow J, Rechenberg W von, Beyer J (1978) Treatment of cryptorchidism with pernasal gonadotropin releasing hormone therapy. Fertil Steril 29:546–551
24. Illig R, Kallmann F, Borkenstein M, Kuber W, Exner GU, Kellerer K, Lunglmayr L, Prader A (1977) Treatment of cryptorchidism by intranasal synthetic luteinizing hormone-releasing hormone. Results of a collaborative double-blind study. Lancet 2:518–520
25. Spona J, Gleispach H, Happ J, Kallmann F, Torresani T, Ohe M von der (1979) Changes of serum testosterone and of LH-RH test after treatment of cyptorchidism by intranasal LH-RH. Endocrinol Exp (Bratisl) 13:204–207
26. Höcht B (1979) Klinische Erfahrungen mit der LH-RH Behandlung beim präpubertalen Maldescensus testis. Habilitationsschrift Universität Würzburg
27. Hadžiselimović F, Girard J, Herzog B, Stalder G (1980) Effect of LH-RH treatment on hypothalamo-pituitary-gonadal axis and Leydig cell ultrastructure in cryptorchid boys. Horm Res 13:358–366
28. Hadžiselimović F, Girard J, Höcht B, Baumann J (1979) Ultrastructure of the cryptorchid Leydig cells after LH-RH treatment. Acta Endocr (Copenh) [Suppl] 225:85
29. Girard J, Baumann J, Ruch W (1980) Diagnostic possibilities in delayed puberty. In: Cacciari E, Prader A (eds) Pathophysiology of puberty. Academic Press, London New York
30. Forest GM, David M, Lecoq A, Jeune M, Bertrams J (1980) Kinetics of the HCG-induced steroidogenic response of the human testis. III. Studies in children of the plasma levels of testosterone and HCG: Rationale for testicular stimulation test. Pediatr Res 14:819–824
31. Forest M, Saez JM (1973) Bertrand J: Assessment of gonadal function in children. Pediatrician 2:102–110

11 Surgical Treatment of Cryptorchidism

J.R. Woodard and T.S. Trulock

11.1 Introduction

Despite the current research and renewed enthusiasm for hormones, surgery remains the cornerstone of therapy for cryptorchidism. Orchiopexy was apparently first attempted by Rosenmerkel in 1820, but the operation did not gain popularity until the end of the nineteenth century when Bevan described the dissection of the cord to provide the length necessary for the testis to reach the scrotum [1, 2]. While there was no provision for anchoring the testis in the scrotum in Bevan's original operation, he later described a purse-string suture at the neck of the scrotum. Subsequently, various methods of testicular fixation have been suggested. Torek advocated fixation of the testis to the fascia lata subcutaneously on the inner aspect of the thigh with a second operation 3 months later to release the testis into the scrotum [3]. Ombredanne anchored the testis by passing it across the scrotal septum to the opposite scrotal compartment [4]. Also popular for a while was the technique of Cabot and Nesbit, where a nonabsorbable suture placed in the lower pole of the testis is brought out through the dependent portion of the scrotum and attached to the inner aspect of the thigh by a rubber band [5]. Lattimer introduced the currently popular technique of placing the testis in a pouch between the dartos and the scrotal skin [6]. However, many surgeons still recommend securing the testis by simply placing a suture through the tunica albuginea, bringing it out through the scrotal skin, and tying it over either a button or dental roll.

Just as there have been a number of different methods for testicular fixation, a variety of surgical approaches have also been advocated. Certainly, the great majority of orchiopexies have been performed through lower quadrant incisions near the groin with extraperitoneal dissection. However, some have advocated

transabdominal, transperitoneal operations as allowing for more thorough abdominal exploration in case of difficulty in locating the testis, as well as for greater ease in bilateral operations [7]. Others recommend a midline vertical incision but a preperitoneal dissection to facilitate delivery of the high undescended testis [8].

11.2 Preoperative Localization of the Testis

True testicular agenesis is rare, occurring bilaterally in 1 of 20,000 and unilaterally in 1 of 5,000 males [9]. In Campbell's series of 12,712 autopsies performed on boys, the testis was reported as unilaterally absent in eight and bilaterally absent in 26 [10]. Anorchism, then, refers to the patient who has a male karyotype and phenotype, but no testicular tissue or Müllerian structures. Jost hypothesized that a testis must have been present during early embryonic development in order to produce normal male external genitalia and to cause regression of the Müllerian structures [11]. The term "vanishing testicle" has been coined to describe this phenomenon [12]. Torsion or vascular occlusion of the neck of the processus vaginalis during descent is thought by many to be the etiology of the vanishing testicle.

Endocrine studies may be useful in evaluating the child with bilaterally non-palpable testes. Levitt et al. suggested that administration of exogenous human chorionic gonadotrophin (HCG) with subsequent monitoring of the serum testosterone level [13]. Patients with normal basal testosterone, LH and FSH who have an increase in serum testosterone after HCG challenge, have functioning testicular tissue and surgical exploration is therefore warranted. Conversely, patients with elevated basal LH and FSH levels and no increase in serum testosterone after HCG challenge have no functioning testicular tissue. If such patients are normal phenotypic males without Müllerian structures, surgical exploration is unnecessary. Unfortunately, there is no endocrine test to evaluate a patient with unilateral cryptorchism.

Several radiological techniques have been utilized to aid in the localization of non-palpable testes. The technique of pneumoperitonography, using nitrous oxide to fill the tunica vaginalis, was described by Lunderquist [14]. Peritonography or herniography, as described by White, was successful in locating a third of nonpalpable testes in the inguinal canal. In addition to a high complication rate, this procedure failed to differentiate monorchism from intraabdominal testes [15]. Transfemoral arteriography has also been used to locate nonpalpable testes, but in young children this procedure is not without risks and may require a general anesthetic. Since flush aortography seldom visualized the spermatic vessels in children, selective gonadal angiograms are necessary. With testicular arterial anatomy being highly variable, selective evaluation often proves impossible. Gonadal venography, a more satisfactory localization technique, is technically simpler and less morbid than arteriography. The left testicular vein is more easily cannulated due to its drainage into the renal vein. Weiss and Glickman reported 43 cases of gonadal venography with minimal complications [16]. In all 11 cases where the gonadal vein terminated into a pampiniform-like plexus, a testis was identified in the same region. When the testicular vein ended blindly, the testis was usually absent.

More recently, computed tomography and ultrasonography have also been used for this purpose. While sonography has successfully localized the testis within the inguinal canal, it has not proved helpful in identifying the site of intra-abdominal testes [17]. CT however, has proved to be considerably more successful in locating nonpalpable testicles either in the abdomen or the canal [18, 19]. There has also been some recent enthusiasm for laparoscopy [20]. However, the role of these newer procedures in the management of patients with cryptorchism, particularly young children, is yet to be defined

Endocrine tests (HCG stimulation) or radiographic evaluation (herniography, arteriography, venography, CT, ultrasound) are not routinely recommended at this time for patients with unilaterally nonpalpable testes. Such patients are best surgically explored through a lower quadrant (inguinal) skin crease incision. The finding of a blind-ending tuft of spermatic vessels, usually adjacent to a blind-ending vas, is diagnostic of monorchism. A blind-ending vas alone is not adequate to make this diagnosis for there may be complete separation of the vas from an abdominal testis. Marshall et al. recently reported such a case in which there was a 7.5 cm separation (nonunion) of the epididymis and the testis [21]. Further exploration is warranted in patients found to have a blind-ending vas but no blind-ending vessels. The importance of locating an abdominal testis is emphasized by a recent report of 13 patients with cryptorchism and malignant testis tumors of whom five had undergone previous limited surgical exploration and were considered to have absent testes [22]. If no testis or tuft of vessels is identified, the peritoneum should be opened and the abdomen explored with the awareness that a high abdominal testis may invaginate the posterior peritoneum and become in effect, an intraperitoneal structure with a mesentery. A unilateral intra-abdominal testis in a postpubertal boy should be removed [23].

11.3 Surgical Techniques

11.3.1 Standard Orchiopexy

The standard orchiopexy technique is applicable to virtually all patients with palpable testes. The objectives of the operation are identification of the testis, gaining adequate length of the spermatic cord, correction of the concommitant hernia, and fixation of the testis within the scrotum (Fig. 1).

A 3.5–4.5 cm incision is made through the lower abdominal skin crease (Fig. 1a). The oblique supra-inguinal incision, used in the adult hernia repair, is cosmetically inferior and should be avoided. Incision of Scarpa's fascia exposes the external oblique aponeurosis. Care must be exercised to avoid injuring a testis located in this superficial inguinal pouch. The external oblique aponeurosis is then split in line with its fibers (Fig. 1b) down through the external inguinal ring using scissors and avoiding injury to the ileoinguinal nerve. Often, the testis is located at the external ring or in the canal, covered by the tunica vaginalis. The attachment of tunica to pubis is divided (Fig. 1c[*]), and with gentle traction on the testis, the cremasteric fibers are dissected from the cord (Fig. 1d). When the cord is adequately skeletonized, the processus vaginalis (hernia sac) can be identified on its anteromedial aspect just distal to the internal inguinal ring. The delicate hernia sac is then separated from the vas and spermatic vessels (Fig. 1e). Some surgeons recommend injecting saline between the hernia sac and the cord structures to facilitate this dissection, but we find this to be unnecessary. When properly isolated, the hernia sac is secured by high ligation with non-absorbable suture (Fig. 1f) and allowed to retract intra-abdominally. If more exposure is required to gain access to the retroperitoneum, the internal oblique muscle is divided upward, beyond the level of the internal ring. At this point, additional length can be obtained by dissecting retroperitoneally and dividing the lateral spermatic fascia (Fig. 1g). This maneuver allows the spermatic vessels to fall medially in a more direct line toward the scrotum. The inferior epigastric vessels (usually one artery and two veins) are divided and the transversalis fascia is opened through the internal ring (Fig. 1h, i), thus providing the testis with a direct route to the scrotum. The tunica vaginalis is then opened distally and the excess sac removed (Fig. 1f). There are several methods of developing a scrotal compartment and anchoring the testis in place. We usually develop a space by inserting the index finger from above (Fig. 1j), then invert the scrotum and wipe off the subcutaneous fat with a gauze sponge. A silk suture is placed through the tunica albuginea of the testis and it is passed through the dependent portion of the scrotum (Fig. 1k, l) and tied over a button or a dental roll (Fig. 1m). There should be no tension on the cord when the testis is anchored thusly in the scrotum. If the subdartos pouch method of fixation is to be used, a 2 cm incision is made in the scrotal skin and a pouch large enough to accomodate the testis is developed between the skin and dartos (Fig. 1n). A clamp is passed through a small opening in the dartos to draw the testis down into the newly created pouch. Extreme care is taken not to twist the spermatic vessels. The tunica vaginalis just above the testis is approximated to the dartos with two sutures, one on

either side (Fig. 1o). The scrotal skin is then closed with chromic catgut horizontal mattress sutures (Fig. 1p). The transversalis fascia and internal oblique muscle are reapproximated lateral to the cord (Fig. 1q) with interrupted non-absorbable sutures, thus creating a new internal ring near the pubis. The external oblique muscle is closed with interrupted non-absorbable sutures (Fig. 1r) and Scarpa's fascia is reapproximated with sutures of either catgut or polyglycolic acid. For optimal cosmetic results, the skin is closed with a subcuticular absorbable suture.

11.3.2 Staged Orchiopexy

The staged orchiopexy (Table 1) for the treatment of the intra-abdominal or high undescended testis was described by Snyder and Chaffin in 1955 and has been advocated by many others [24]. Gross and Jewett found that a second operation was required to achieve a scrotal testis in only 8 of 1,222 patients [25]. For Persky and Albert, however, 13 of 400 patients required a second operation and in 9 of these 13 the testis was successfully relocated at the second procedure [26]. The remaining for patients required orchiectomy. Firor found staged procedures to be more frequently necessary with 21.5% of his 287 patients requiring

Table 1. Results of staged orchiopexy

References	No. cases	Successful result No. (%)
Snyder and Chaffin (1955) [24]	7	6 (86)
Gross and Replogle (1963) [44]	24	24 (100)
Bill and Shanahan (1964) [45]	2	2 (100)
Williams and Burkholder (1963) [46]	3 (prune belly)	3 (100)
Lynn (1969) [47]	2	2 (100)
Persky and Albert (1971) [26]	13	9 (70)
Firor (1971) [27]	32	30 (94)
Corkery (1975) [30]	5	5 (100)
Zer et al. (1975) [28]	62	48 (77)
Kiesewetter et al. (1981) [29]	60	56 (93)
	210	185 (80)

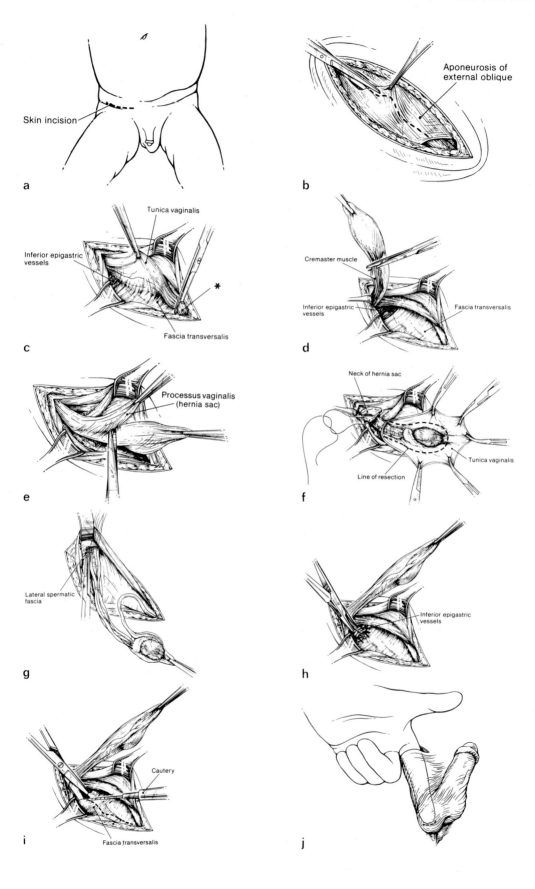

a   Skin incision

b   Aponeurosis of external oblique

c   Tunica vaginalis
    Inferior epigastric vessels
    Fascia transversalis
    *

d   Cremaster muscle
    Inferior epigastric vessels
    Fascia transversalis

e   Processus vaginalis (hernia sac)

f   Neck of hernia sac
    Line of resection
    Tunica vaginalis

g   Lateral spermatic fascia

h   Inferior epigastric vessels

i   Cautery
    Fascia transversalis

j

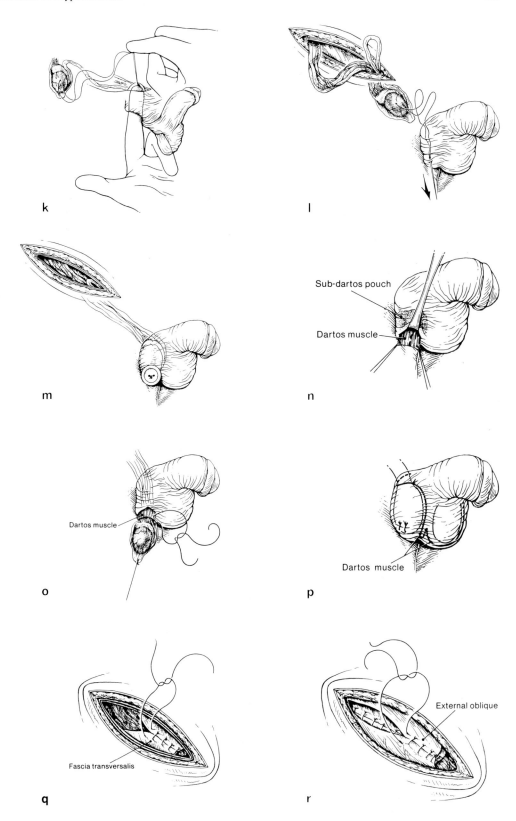

Fig. 1a–r. Steps of incision in staged orchiopexy (*) attachment of tunica to pubis.

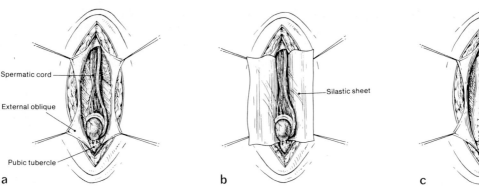

Fig. 2a–c. Fixation of testis in staged orchiopexy

a second procedure [27]. In 1975, Zer reported 62 cases of planned staged orchiopexies [28]. Satisfactory placement of the testis in the scrotum was achieved in 90% of his patients. In only two was an atrophic testis found at the second operation and these authors recommended waiting 3 years between procedures. Kieswetter et al. recently reported experience with 60 staged procedures in which the success rate was 82% [29].

Most surgeons encounter difficulty in the dissection of the testis and cord during the second procedure. Corkery described a technique to facilitate that dissection while protecting the testis and the cord from injury [30]. He recommended wrapping the cord and testis in a silicone sheath at the initial operation. At the time of re-exploration, the silicone sheath is removed and the testis is placed safely in the scrotum. In a review highly critical of staged orchiopexy, Redman suggested that the satisfactory results reported were due to an inadequate initial operation and that there was no documentation of further elongation of the spermatic cord after reoperation [31].

The technique for the initial stage is similar to the standard orchiopexy previously described (Fig. 1). A lower abdominal skin crease incision is made, the cord is mobilized, and the hernia is corrected. All maneuvers previously described to obtain cord length and the most direct route to the scrotum are utilized. Depending on the length of the cord, the testis is anchored to the pubis (Fig. 2a), the inguinal ligament, or the upper portion of the scrotum. Excess tension on the cord, which might result in testicular atrophy, should be avoided. In the Corkery operation, after adequate mobilization

the cord and testis are wrapped in a silastic membrane. The silastic sheath is placed around the cord and testis (Fig. 2b) and sewn into a pouch with a continuous silk suture (Fig. 2c). A small opening is left in the distal aspect of this pouch allowing the lower pole of the testis to be anchored to the pubis.

After an interval of a year, the second-stage procedure is performed through the original skin incision. The external oblique aponeurosis, identified by the presence of silk sutures, is opened with extreme care. The cord is then dissected free up to the internal ring. The anatomy is often obscured by scar formation, making this dissection tedious. It is at this point that injury to the vessels or vas is most likely. If further length is required, the vas and vessels should be dissected in the retroperitoneal space. The testis is then placed in the scrotum and anchored by one of the previously described methods. The testis must be under no tension.

11.3.3 Fowler-Stephens (Long-Loop Vas) Orchiopexy

For the surgeon faced with a high undescended testis, the technique of vascular pedicle division, popularized by Fowler and Stephens [32] is becoming an increasingly attractive alternative to staged orchiopexy (Table 2). While the concept of spermatic vessel transsection was first described by Bevan in 1903, early results with the procedure were poor and it quickly fell into disfavor [33]. Interest was renewed in 1959 when Fowler and Stephens described the vascular anatomy of the undescended testis. Using operative testicular angiography, they demonstrated vascular anastomoses between the vasal and the spermatic arteries. To assure the adequacy of blood supply from the vasal artery, these authors recommended that the spermatic vessels be temporarily occluded and that the tunica albuginea then be incised and observed for fresh bleeding. Using this technique, Fowler and Stephens achieved good results with their procedure in 8 of 12 patients. In 1967, Brendler and Wulfson reported five cases using a similar technique, all with good results [34]. These authors emphasized two additional important technical points: there should be no dissection within the substance of the cord, and the spermatic vessels should be divided well above the point where the vas and the vessels meet.

In 1972, Clatworthy and his associates reported on 32 Fowler-Stephens operations among 342 orchiopexies [35]. They divided their patients into two groups. In the first group, the operation was done as a "premeditated", primary procedure. In the second group, the operation was resorted to as a "salvage" procedure following an extensive dissection of the cord. In the premeditated group, a successful result (no testicular atrophy) was obtained in 18 of 21 patients. In the second group, where vessel division was performed after extensive dissection of the cord, only 6 of 11 operations were successful. To preserve the vital collateral circulation, these authors recommended leaving the floor of the canal and the inferior epigastric vessel intact, sparing the vessels in the area of the gubernaculum, and avoiding mobilization of the posterior wall of the hernia sac. This latter point was also emphasized by Johnston, who in reference to orchiopexy in the prune-belly syndrome recommended leaving a wide strip of peritoneum attached to the vas to protect the delicate vasal vessels [36].

Gibbons et al. used the Fowler-Stephens technique in 17 of 30 patients with intra-abdominal testes [37]. Postoperative atrophy occurred in 5 of 17 (30%), 4 of whom had prune-belly syndrome. These authors retrospectively analyzed the possible errors in the Fowler-Stephens orchiopexy as (1) failure to leave a wide strip of peritoneum overlying the vas, (2) attempting to salvage a scrotal placement after cord mobilization and dissection, (3) ligation of the spermatic cord too close to the testis, and (4) direct injury to the vasal artery.

Table 2. Fowler-Stephens orchiopexy

Authors	Testes	Failure	Success
Moschcowitz [48]	22	1	21
Mixter [49]	15	13	2
MacCollum [50]	5	5	0
Fowler and Stephens [51]	12	4	8
Jones [52]	17	8	9
Brendler and Wulfson [34]	5	0	5
Datta et al. [53]	3	0	3
Clatworthy et al. [35]	32	8	24
Gibbons et al. [37]	27	5	22
	138	44 (32%)	94 (68%)

Conditions which preclude a Fowler-Stephens orchiopexy are (1) testis with a short vas, making scrotal placement, even after ligation of the spermatic vessels, impossible, (2) hypoplastic testes with uncertain vascular supply, (3) segmental vasal atresia, and (4) a detached epididymis.

The operation is performed through a skin crease incision that is perhaps slightly longer than for a standard orchiopexy. After the inguinal canal is opened in the standard manner, the internal oblique muscle is divided superiorly and laterally to gain greater retroperitoneal exposure. The hernia sac is identified and opened anteriorly. The vas can be seen looping down the posteromedial wall of the hernia sac and returning superiorly to the epididymis and testis. While the hernia sac is dissected away form the testicular vessels well above the gonad, it is allowed to remain adherent to the vas. After the hernia sac has been closed with a silk purse-string suture, a Fowler-Stephens "test" is carried out by placing a vascular bulldog clamp on the spermatic vessels (Fig. 3) about 5 cm above the gonad. The color of the testis is observed for several minutes after which a small incision is made in the tunica albuginea. If brisk red bleeding occurs, and continues for several minutes, the collateral circulation is considered to be adequate and the spermatic vessels can be ligated and divided. The tunica albuginea incision can be closed with a small catgut suture. Some increased length can be obtained by incising the posterior wall of the residual hernia sac, but care must be taken to divide as few of the small vascular arcades as possible

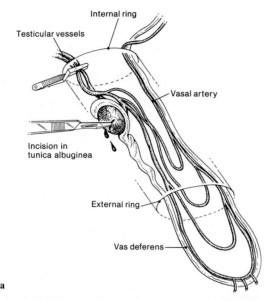

a

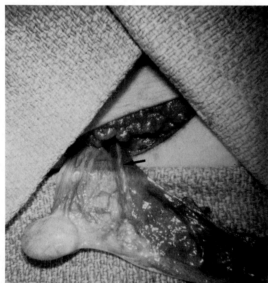

b

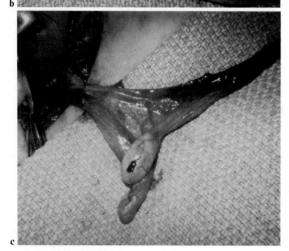

c

and yet allow placement of the testis in the scrotum. Fixation of the testis in the scrotum is done in the standard manner. Postoperative swelling is usually considerably more than that seen with the standard orchiopexy.

11.3.4 Microsurgical (Autotransplantation) Technique

Recent advances in the use of the operative microscope have made possible the anastomosis of vessels 1/3 mm in diameter. These techniques, pioneered in the animal laboratory, are rapidly gaining the enthusiasm of urologists. Initially, urologic microsurgery was confined primarily to reanastomosis of the vas deferens to restore fertility after vasectomy. The same techniques now provide a method of maintaining arterial supply and venous drainage to the testis during orchiopexy. The first successful orchiopexies using microvascular techniques were reported by Silber and Kelly in 1976 [38]. Martin and Salibian accomplished orchiopexies in two patients in whom arterial supply and venous drainage were maintained using microsurgical techniques [39]. Patency was verified in one of their patients by use of arteriography and radionucleide scan. Romas and associates reported using microvascular techniques in four intra-abdominal testes [40]. Atrophy did not occur in any of the four testes, but, due to inadequate cord length, one testis was placed at the level of the external ring. In the series of Mac-Mahon et al. two of eight operations resulted in testicular atrophy, and while Wacksman et al. reported successful microvascular orchiopexy in four patients, no mention was made of postoperative follow-up [41, 42].

Although these initial reports of microsurgical orchiopexy are impressive, the role of microsurgery is still to be established. With precise technique, a similarly high success rate may be approachable with division of the spermatic

Fig. 3. a The collateral circulation between the vasal and testicular vessels. A bulldog vascular clamp has been applied to the testicular vessels and the tunica albuginea has been incised to demonstrate adequate blood supply. b The long-loop vas with collateral vessels between the distal vas and testicular vessels. *Arrow* indicates vas. c Fresh arterial bleeding from incised testis with bulldog vascular clamp on the testicular vessels

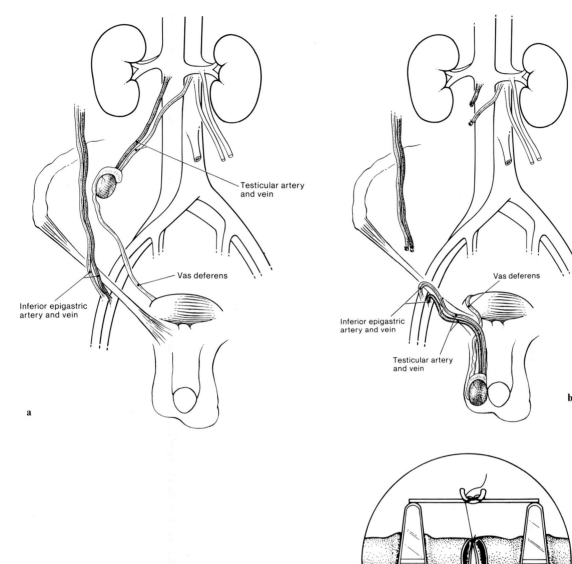

Fig. 4. a Intra-abdominal testis showing short testicular artery and vein in relation to inferior epigastric artery and vein. b The testicular artery and vein have been ligated and transected, as have the inferior epigastric artery and vein. The testicular vessels have been anastomosed to the inferior epigastric vessels and the testis placed in a sub-dartos pouch in the scrotum. c Ackland clamp used to approximate testicular and inferior epigastric vessels

vessels and no microsurgical reconstruction (Fowler-Stephens). The latter procedure will probably remain that used by most surgeons because of the simpler technique, shorter operating time, and high success rate. With the small numbers of cases suitable for the microsurgical technique, it is likely that these operations will remain in the domain of relatively few urologic surgeons.

For microvascular transplantation (Fig. 4), a high oblique abdominal incision is used, with care not to injure the inferior epigastric vessels. The abdominal musculature is divided with electric cautery and the testis is located with a combination of retroperitoneal and intraperitoneal dissection. Once identified, the spermatic vessels are traced to the aorta and vena cava (Fig. 4a). Magnification with optical loops aids

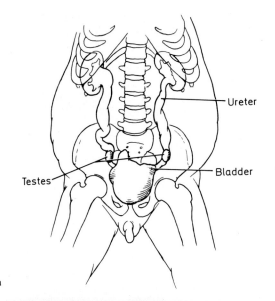

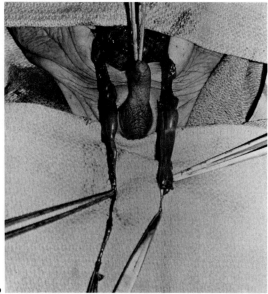

Fig. 5. a Typical position of intra-abdominal testes in patients with prune-belly syndrome. Testes are on posterior pelvic wall overlying ureters. **b** Transabdominal orchiopexy in neonate with prune-belly syndrome. Testes were mobilized along with urinary tract reconstruction and can be seen to easily reach level of scrotum with vascular pedicles intact

allows exposure of the inferior epigastric vessels, which are carefully dissected superiorly and divided under the rectus muscle to assure adequate length. The proximal ends of these vessels are occluded with microvascular clips. The spermatic vessels are now divided and attention is directed to the microvascular anastomosis (Fig. 4b). Since the spermatic artery is smaller than the inferior epigastric, it will require spatulation for satisfactory anastomosis. The internal spermatic vein, which is larger than the artery, is anastomosed first. Magnification ×25 is required. Ends of the veins are placed in a microvascular clamp and interrupted sutures of 10-0 or 11-0 nylon on a BV-6 or St-7 needle are used. A similar technique is used for the arterial anastomosis. Although perfusion of the testis during the ischemic period is unnecessary, cooling may be helpful and systemic heparin therapy is recommended by some. With the vascular anastomosis completed (Fig. 4c), the testis is placed in a dartos pouch. There must be no tension on the anastomosis. The abdominal wall is closed cautiously to avoid damaging or angulating the internal spermatic vessels. Postoperatively, the patency of the anastomosis may be verified by arteriography or a radionuclide scan.

11.3.5 Neonatal Transabdominal Orchiopexy

In patients born with the prune belly syndrome, one expects intra-abdominal testes (Fig. 5a) without the potential for spontaneous descent. It has been demonstrated that these testes can be brought successfully into the scrotum with their vascular pedicle intact by means of a transabdominal, transperitoneal orchiopexy carried out during the first weeks of life, either in conjunction with urinary tract reconstruction or as a primary procedure (Fig. 5b) [43]. The spermatic cord is mobilized transperitoneally to the origin of the spermatic vein and artery, after which the testis is passed through the abdominal wall at the site of the external inguinal ring and into the scrotum, where it is anchored with a button as described in the standard orchiopexy. We have had success with this operation on at least one side in 12 consecutive prune-belly patients. It might very well be that other individuals with intra-abdominal testes would be amenable to more successful surgery if per-

in this dissection. The spermatic vessels are divided near their origin and tagged with fine nylon sutures. The vas deferens is dissected downward to the bladder. Collateral circulation to the testis from the vasal vessels must be preserved, just as in the Fowler-Stephens operation. Incision of the floor of the inguinal canal

formed during the neonatal period. Unfortunately, with the exception of babies with prune-belly syndrome, those who might benefit from this early, aggressive approach cannot easily be identified.

With the technical expertise now available, it is possible to achieve scrotal position in almost any patient with an undescended testis. However, we must continue to refine our criteria for determining which testes are worthy of orchiopexy. The indications and contraindications for orchiopexy are still to be generally agreed upon.

References

1. Rosenmerkel JF (1820) Über die Radikalkur des in der Weiche liegenden Testikels bei nicht erfolgtem Descensus desselben. J Lindauer, Munich
2. Bevan AD (1899) Operation for undescended testicle and congenital inguinal hernia. JAMA 33:773
3. Torek F (1909) The technic of orchiopexy. NY J Med 90:948
4. Ombredanne L (1927) Sur l'orchiopexie. Bull Soc Pédiatr Paris 25:473
5. Cabot H, Nesbit RM (1931) Undescended testis. Arch Surg 22:850
6. Lattimer JK (1957) Scrotal pouch technique for orchiopexy. J Urol 78:628
7. Flinn RA, King LR (1971) Experiences with the midline transabdominal approach in orchiopexy. Surg Gynecol Obstet 133:285
8. Hunt JB, Withington R, Smith AM (1981) The midline preperitoneal approach to orchiopexy. Am Surg 47:184
9. Burrow M, Gough MH (1970) Bilateral absence of testes. Lancet 1:366
10. Campbell MF (1970) Anomalies of the genital tract. In: Campbell MF, Harrison JH (eds) Urology. Saunders, Philadelphia, p 1625
11. Jost A (1953) Problems of fetal endocrinology. Rec Prog Horm Res 8:379
12. Abeyarotine MC, Aherne WA, Scott JES (1969) The vanishing testis. Lancet 2:822
13. Levitt SB, Kogan SJ, Engel RM, Weiss RM, Martin DC, Ehrlich RM (1978) The impalpable testis: a rational approach to management. J Urol 120:515
14. Lunderquist A, Rafstedt S (1967) Roentgenologic diagnosis of cryptorchidism. J Urol 98:219
15. White JJ, Haller JA Jr, Dorst JP (1970) Congenital inguinal hernia and inguinal herniography. Surg Clin North Am 50:823
16. Weiss RM, Glickman MG, Lytton B (1977) Venographic localization of the non-palpable undescended testis in children. J Urol 117:513
17. Madrazo BL, Klugo RC, Parks JA, Diloreto R (1979) Ultrasonographic demonstration of undescended testes. Radiology 133:181
18. Lee JKT, McClennan BC, Stanley RJ, Sagel SS (1980) Utility of computed tomography in the localization of the undescended testis. Radiology 135:121
19. Wolverson MK, Jagannadharao B, Sundarm M, Riaz MA, Nalesnik WJ, Houttuin E (1980) CT in localization of impalpable cryptorchid testes. Am J Roentgenol 134:725
20. Silber SJ, Cohen R (1980) Laparoscopy for cryptorchidism. J Urol 124:928
21. Marshall FF, Weissman RM, Jeffs RD (1980) Cryptorchidism: The surgical implications of non-union of the epididymis and testis. J Urol 125:560
22. Brothers LR III, Weber CH Jr, Bull TR Jr (1978) Anorchism versus cryptorchism: The importance of a diligent search for intra-abdominal testis. J Urol 119:707
23. Martin DC, Menck HR (1975) The undescended testis: management after puberty. J Urol 114:77
24. Snyder WH Jr, Chaffin L (1955) Surgical management of undescended testes. Report of 363 cases. JAMA 157:129
25. Gross RE, Jewett TC (1956) Surgical experiences from 1,222 operations for undescended testes. JAMA 160:634
26. Persky L, Albert DJ (1971) Staged orchiopexy. Surg Gynecol Obstet 132:43
27. Firor HV (1971) Two-stage orchiopexy. Arch Surg 102:598
28. Zer M, Wooloch Y, Dintsman M (1975) Staged orchiorhaphy. Therapeutic procedure in cryptorchid testicle with a short spermatic cord. Arch Surg 110:387
29. Kiesewetter WB, Mammen K, Kalyglou M (1981) The rationale and results in two-stage orchiopexies. J Pediatr Surg [Suppl] 16:631
30. Corkery JJ (1975) Staged orchiopexy – a new technique. J Pediatr Surg 10:515
31. Redman JF (1977) The staged orchiopexy: a critical review of the literature. J Urol 117:113
32. Fowler R, Stephens FO (1959) The role of testicular vascular anatomy in the salvage of high undescended testes. Aust NZ J Surg 29:92
33. Bevan AD (1903) The surgical treatment of undescended testicle: A further contribution. JAMA 41:718
34. Brendler H, Wulfson MA (1967) Surgical treatment of high undescended testis. Surg Gynec and Obst 124:605
35. Clatworthy HW Hr, Hollanbaugh RS, Grosfeld JL (1972) The "long loop vas" orchiopexy for high undescended testis. Amer Surg 38:69
36. Johnston JH: Prune Belly syndrome (1977) In: Eckstein HB, Huhenfellner R, Williams DI (eds) Surgical Pediatric Urology. Philadelphia, Saunders WB Co., p 240
37. Gibbons MD, Cromie WJ, Duckett JW Jr (1979) Management of the abdominal undescended testicle. J Urol 122:76
38. Silber SJ, Kelly J (1976) Successful autotransplantation of an intra-abdominal testis to the scrotum by microvascular technique. J Urol 115:452
39. Martin DC, Salibian A (1980) Orchiopexy utilizing microvascular surgical techniques. J Urol 123:263
40. Romas NA, Janecka I, Krisiloff M (1978) Role of microsurgery in orchiopexy. Urology 12:670
41. MacMahon RA, O'Brien B McC, Cussen JL (1976) The use of microsurgery in the treatment of the undescended testis. J Ped Surg 11:521
42. Wacksman J, Dinner M, Straffon RP (1980) Technique of testicular autotransplantation using a microvascular anastomosis. Surg Gyn and Obst 150:399
43. Woodard JR, Parrott TS (1978) Orchiopexy in the prune belly syndrome. Br J Urol 50:348

44. Gross RE, Replogle RL (1963) Treatment of the undescended testis. Opinions gained from 1,767 operations. Postgrad Med 34:266
45. Bill AH Jr, Shanahan DA (1964) The management of undescended testicle. Surg Clin North Am 44:1571
46. Williams DI, Burkholder GV (1967) The prune belly syndrome. J Urol 98:244
47. Lynn HB (1969) Undescended testis. Can Family Physician 15:33
48. Moschcowitz AV (1910) The anatomy and treatment of undescended testis: With especial reference to the Bevan operation. Ann Surg 52:821
49. Mixter CG (1924) Undescended testicle: Operative treatment and end-results. Surg Gynecol Obstet 39:275
50. MacCollum DW (1935) Clinical study of the spermatogenesis of undescended testicles. Arch Surg 31:290
51. Fowler R Jr, Stephens FD (1963) The role of testicular vascular anatomy in the salvage of high undescended testes. In: Webster R (ed) Congenital malformations of the rectum, anus, and genito-urinary tracts. E & S Livingstone Ltd, London, pp 306–320
52. Jones PG (1966) Undescended testes. Aust Paediatr J 2:36
53. Datta NS, Tanaka T, Zinner NR, Mishkin FS (1977) Division of spermatic vessels in orchiopexy: Radionuclide evidence of preservation of testicular circulation. J Urol 118:447

12 Conclusions

F. Hadžiselimović

Testicular descent is an event typical among mammalian species. It is observable only in mammals living on the ground and represents a parallel form of evolutionary development. Generally, the mammalian species which have testicular descent are also evolutionarily younger. Three different types of gonad position can be distinguished:

1. Naturally cryptorchid (testicond)
2. Incomplete descent (partial descent; only the epididymis has descended)
3. Complete descent (testes and epididymis have descended)

12.1 The Role of the Epididymis in Testicular Descent

The *epididymis* has a prime role in testicular descent because:

1. The epididymis always precedes the testes during descent and the gubernaculum is never in direct contact with the testis.
2. The differentiation of the epididymis starts at the cranial pole and is completed when testicular descent is terminated.
3. Testicular descent does not take place if there is a dissociation of the epididymis and the testis.
4. In newborn boys suffering from cryptorchidism, the epididymis has a wide interstitium and less tubuli, indicating that its development is impaired.

It is evident from our results that the caput epididymidis has important function in achieving testicular descent (a constant impression at the cranial testis pole is observable as a result of the pressure developed from the caput epididymidis during descent). Cauda and corpus epididymidis also participate in testicular descent but the degree of interaction is still to be estimated.

Experimentally, the application of estradiol during gestation induces in all male mice issues a testicular testosterone deficit and hinders the development and differentiation of the Wolffian duct, thus resulting in cryptorchidism. Both GnRH treatment and HCG treatment induce in cryptorchid rats and mice the development of Leydig cells and an increase of testosterone production. The high local testosterone concentration influences further epididymis development and consequently descent takes place. The gubernaculum mainly acts as a guide in testicular descent; aberrant insertion of the gubernaculum results in ectopic testes. The processus vaginalis and a normally developed inguinal canal are the prerequisites for descent the former one can be described as a facilitator for testis descent during its passage through the inguinal canal.

12.2 Clinical and Pathophysiological Implications in Cryptorchid Boys

Important *primary pathological changes* in the human testes are observable immediately after birth within the interstitium of cryptorchid boys. The Leydig cells show typical signs of atrophy. In the period between 4 weeks and 3 months of life, hypertrophy and hyperplasia of the Leydig cells, as a consequence of increased gonadotropin secretion, are lacking in cryptorchid testes. This corresponds to the endocrinological findings published in the literature of impaired testosterone secretion in cryptorchid infants and normal secretion in those with late testicular descent. The *atrophy* of the Leydig cells is permanently observable throughout childhood the cryptorchid patients. This appears prominent the more hypogonadotropic the patients is. This atrophy is due to impaired intrauterine gonadotropin stimulation. It was encountered in 80% of cryptorchid boys during childhood. However the expressivity of this deficiency varies considerably. It underlines the hormonal imbalance as a main cause of this malformation. The remaining 20% of cryptorchid boys represent a heterogenous group with differing morphological and histological abnormalities. In true cryptorchid testes up till puberty, there is no transformation of A spermatogonia into B spermatogonia. This contrasts to the iatrogenic cryptorchid testes in which the hypothalamo-pituitary-gonadal axis is normal and the Leydig cells are normally developed. Here, the transformation of A spermatogonia into B spermatogonia and subsequently into spermatocytes takes place.

The *secondary pathologic changes* due to an unfavorable position begin as early as the 2nd year of life. The thickening of the peritubular connective tissue is significant in the 3rd year of life and reaches its peak about the 7th year of life. The collagenization of the interstitium in cryptorchid testes which starts in the 2nd year progresses until puberty. This collagenization, present in both true and jatrogenic cryptorchid testes, is a mucopolysaccharide barrier preventing adequate perfusion of the seminiferous tubuli and induces their atrophic changes.

The fact that cryptorchid boys are similar to boys with normal descent in terms of number of germ cells until the 6th month of life, undoubtedly speaks against the concept of inherently "sick" testes.

Testicular *tumors* are rare. Their peak incidence occurs between the ages of 25 and 35 years. A single value determined for the risk of malignant disease in patients with cryptorchidism was 48.91 per 100,000, which represents a 22.23-fold increase compared with those individuals with scrotal testes. The incidence of malignant neoplasm in this latter group was 2.2 per 100,000. An intra-abdominal cryptorchid testis further increases the risk of testicular tumor. The increased occurrence of testicular tumors in cryptorchid patients is hypothesized to be caused (a) by prenatally created congenital anomalies and (b) by postnatal carcinogenic agents responsible for development of atrophy.

The vast majority of cryptorchid testes (more than 60%) are within the inguinal canal, mainly around the external inguinal pouch. Untreated

bilateral cryptorchid patients have a sterility rate of over 90%. The unilateral cryptorchid untreated patients are infertile in 50.6% and subfertile in 28.8% of cases. Even if the testes are prescrotal, histological alterations are evident and with increasing age become more prominent.

The earlier in life the scrotal position is achieved, the better the chances of achieving fertility. There is no doubt today that the cryptorchid testes should be in the scrotal position before the 2nd year of life.

The treatment of first choice is hormonal therapy. GnRH *treatment* alone has a success rate of 60%. It should be stressed that Leydig cells are also recruited in unsuccessfully treated patients, enabling additional low doses of HCG to develop their influence successfully. Therefore if no success is forthcoming, an additional weekly dosage of 1,500 IU HCG is recommended for a further 3 weeks immediately after cessation of GnRH treatment. The success rate immediately after cessation of combined treatment is 80%. The best results are achieved if the testes are originally located in an inguinal or suprascrotal position.

A relapse has been observed in 14.5% of hormonally treated patients 6 months after cessation of therapy. In these cases additional GnRH treatment should be undertaken. All children successfully treated either hormonally or surgically have to be checked annually until puberty; relapse is still possible 2 years after cessation of treatment.

Should hormonal therapy fail, immediate and early orchiopexy is advisable in bilateral prepubertal cryptorchidism and in most unilateral cases. No treatment is advisable in boys who have severe mental defects or have major genetic disorders. Orchiectomy may be the treatment of choice for many unilateral intra-abdominal testes and for the symptomatic inguinal testis or bilateral testes after puberty. Surgery should be performed by an experienced specialist.

However, the question of whether early treatment would preserve fertility in all cryptorchid boys remains to be solved. Particularly in regard to the 20% of cryptorchid boys with a marked gonadotropin deficiency, any such assertion should be greeted with scepticism.

13 Treatment Schedule

F. Hădziselimović

1. All newborn males should be screened to ascertain if any signs of cryptorchidism are present.
2. Any male suspected of being cryptorchid at birth should have his plasma testosterone examined between 2 and 6 months of age.
3. Early GnRH treatment (after the age of 10 months) should be commenced.
4. A daily dose of 3×400 µg GnRH nasal spray should be administered for 4 weeks.
5. If no success is forthcoming, an additional weekly dose of 1,500 IU HCG is recommended for a further 3 weeks.
6. In cases of relapses of hormonal treatment an additional 4 weeks of GnRH treatment is recommended.
7. If a concomitant hernia or a true ectopia is encountered, surgery is the treatment of first choice.
8. If the treatment fails, surgery should be performed by an experienced surgeon prior the child's second birthday.
9. All boys treated should have an annual check-up until they reach the age of puberty.
10. To determine the position of the testes accurately, the child should be seated in a cross-legged position when examined.
11. If the cryptorchid child is mentally retarded, the related syndromes should be excluded.

14 Prospectives

F. Hadžiselimović and B. Höcht

The cardinal question remains: Will the prognosis of fertility improve if a cryptorchid testis is treated before the age of 2 years in those boys with severe hypogonadotrophic hypogonadism?

If the biopsies of the cryptorchid boys taken $1^1/_2$ years after orchydopexic are compared to those obtained at the time of the orchydopexy no increase in the number of germ cells are discernible [1]. Thirty percent of cryptorchid boys, lacking germ cells at the time of the operation, are sterile despite successful treatment [2]. This questions the preliminary results of other findings [3] and indicates that a functioning hypothalamo-pituitary-gonadal axis is a prerequisite for normal germ cell development. Two patients aged 3 and 9 years, suffering respectively from bilateral cryptorchidism (F.P., Würzburg) and unilateral cryptorchidism with hydrocele and inguinal hernia on the contralateral descended side (U.M., Basel), were treated. Their S/T index was: F.P., left testis 0.1, right testis 0.08; U.M., left testis 0.08 (Fig. 1). The severity of gonadal damage in both boys indicates that they belong to the group of cryptorchid patients where sterility or severe impairment of fertility will develop after puberty. After discussing the treatment schedule with the ethical committee, the parents were informed about the mode of treatment and the necessity of a testicular biopsy after treatment was discontinued. Although the gonads were severely impaired the basal FSH and LH values were normal, indicating hypogonadotrophic hypogonadism. The testosterone plasma values were also within the normal range. Following intranasal application of 10 μg GnRH$_a$, peak LH and FSH plasma values were achieved after a 4 h period [4]. The treatment schedule was: one squirt of GnRH$_a$ 10 μg applied nasally every 48 h for 5 (F.P.) and 6 (U.M.) months. The clinical check-ups were performed every 2nd week. To check the function of the pituitary, blood was sampled monthly before and 4 h after 10 μg GnRH$_a$ nasal spray application. Testosterone, LH and FSH were estimated by RIA. After the cessation of therapy, a right testicular biopsy in the 3-year-old bilateral cryptorchid boy (F.P.) and a bilateral testicular biopsy in the 9-year-old boy (U.M.) were performed (Fig. 1). In order to estimate the germ cell number, at least 50 seminiferous tubules

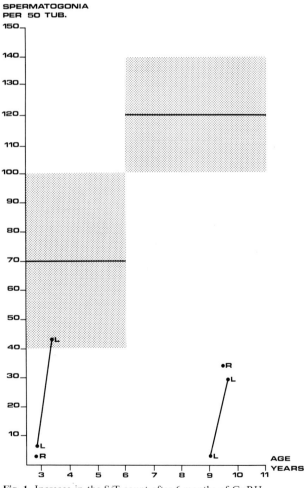

Fig. 1. Increase in the S/T count after 6 months of GnRH$_a$ treatment. *Shaded area,* normal range of spermatogonia

were counted. On the day before surgery, an additional GnRH stimulation test (100 µg GnRH i.v.) was performed.

The treatment with GnRH$_a$ induced no secondary sexual changes for the whole period of the treatment. The penis length remained unchanged. No relevant testicular enlargement was noted. At the beginning of the treatment both patients had soft palpating testes. Three months after commencement the testes had improved considerably in their consistency. The substitution of 10 µg GnRH$_a$ increased the germ cell number significantly (Fig. 1). There was also an increase in the tubulus diameter of patient U.M. and a development of the juvenile Leydig cells in both patients. No downregulation of the pituitary was observable during the whole period of treatment. The LH and FSH basal and peak plasma values, as well as basal testosterone plasma values, remained unchanged during the whole treatment.

Substituting low doses of GnRH$_a$ every other day to achieve the increase of the germ cells is considered unique even today, and promises a completely new approach to the treatment of cryptorchidism in particular and hypogonadism in general. Further investigations in this field should confirm the initial encouraging results and open new horizons.

References

1. Sizonenko CP, Schindler AM, Cuendet A (1981) Clinical evaluation and management of testicular disorders before puberty. In: Burger H, Kretser D de (eds) The testis. Raven Press, New York
2. Canlorbe P (1966) Les cryptorchidies (étude de 145 cas). Ann de Pédiatrie 16:249–278
3. Ludwig G, Potempa J (1975) Der optimale Zeitpunkt der Behandlung des Kryptorchismus. Dtsch Med Wochenschr 100:680–683
4. Ohe M von der: Wissenschaftliche Monographie. Kryptocur Höchst Frankfurt a.M. 1982

Subject Index

Page numbers in **bold face** refer to figures

Ad spermatogonium **14**, 35
androgen, mechanism of action 62
anorchism, endocrine studies 98, 115
Ap spermtogonium **14**, 35
atypical germ cells 55, **57**, 86
autotransplantation 122

B spermatogonium **14**, 36

carcinoma in situ **56**, 86
 ultrastructure 55
choriocarcinoma 87
conus inguinalis 3, 23
cryptorchid epididymis **31**, **32**
 histology 28
 interstitium 30
cryptorchid testis
 abdominally located 93
 Ad spermatogonia 48
 Ap spermatogonia 48, **49**
 binuclear spermatogonia 48
 development 45
 fetal spermatogonia 48
 inguinal 47
 inguinally located 93
 intra-abdominal 47
 Leydig cells 52, **54**
 morphometry 45
 number of spermatogonia 45
 peritubular connective tissue 50, **52**
 Sertoli cells 50
 superficial inguinal pouch 47
 suprascrotally located 93
 transitional spermatogonia 48, **49**
 tubulus diameter 45
 ultrastructure 48
 volume of tubules 45
cryptorchidism
 androgen deficiency 26, 65, 66
 chromosomal anomalies **94**
 concomitant findings 94
 dihydrotestosterone 26, 62, 63, 64
 estrogen-induced 25
 fertility 71
 immunology 76
 incidence 93
 Leydig cell atrophy 25, **54**
 spontaneous congenital 26
 testicular testosterone 25
cryptorchidism theory, Gestaltungstheorie 4
 gubernaculum swelling 5

intersex 4
intra-abdominal pressure 6
meander-shaped gubernaculum 5
mechanical barrier 6
musculus cremaster 5
pelvic rotation 6
thermoregulatory 4

descended testis, contralateral lesion 75
diethylstilbestrol 84

ectopic testis 93
embryonal cell Ca 87
epididymal descent 7, **18**
epididymis 23
 role 23, 127
examination technique 95

fertility
 bilateral pathologic process 80
 in compensatory testicular hypertrophy 74
fertility data
 analysis 73
 HCG-induced descent 73
fetal spermatogonium 13, 14, **14**, 35
α-fetoprotein 95
Fowler-Stephens orchiopexy 120, **121**
FSH, impaired increase 67

genital malformations 95
genital tract
 differentiation 11
 indifferent stage 11
germ cells 12
 development 14
 transformation 14
gliding testis 93
GnRH
 gonadotropin profile **102**, **103**
 pharmacokinetic studies 104
GnRH treatment 101
 antibodies 113
 FMV urine **107**
 cryptorchid mice 26
 gonadotropin values **107**
 histological changes 106, 107
 Leydig cells 106, **108**, **109**, **110**
 morphological abnormalities 112
 precursor Leydig cells 106

GnRH treatment
  randomized study 107
  relapse 113
  Sertoli cells **111**
  side effects 113
  success rate 112
GnRH$_a$ treatment 131, 132
gonadal venography 116
gonocyte **13**, **14**
  development 35
  type 1 **13**
  type 2 **13**
  ultrastructure 12
gubernaculum **22**, 23

HCG response, in cryptorchid boys 66
HCG treatment 101
heredity 94
hernias malformations 95
herniography 116
HLA-Dw7 85
hypothalamo-pituitary-gonadal axis 59
  in cryptorchid boys 65
  development **60**
  feedback mechanism 60
  testing 64

iatrogenic cryptorchidism 53, 55, 128
infertility
  age at treatment 71
  definition 72
  factor 71
  patient source 71
injury from surgery 72

juvenile Leydig cells **41**

Leydig cell
  fetal 15, **16**
  juvenile **110**
  precursor **108**
  testosterone production 61
  transitional stage **109**
LH deficiency 66

male duct differentiation 17
malignant degeneration
  etiology 83
  germinal atrophy 83
  hormonal imbalance 83
  risk 83
  temperature 83
  trauma 83
menarche 85
mesenchymal cord 11
mesonephros 17
Müllerian duct 17, 64
mumps orchitis 85
myofibroblasts **22**, 35, **43**, 50

normal testis, in puberty 35

orchiectomy 128
orchiopexy, neonatal transabdominal 124

penis, length **96**
peritubular connective tissue **43**, 50
pneumoperitonography 116
postoperative atrophy 121
premalignant changes 86
primary sex cords 11
primordial germ cells 12, 55
processus vaginalis **18**, **19**, **20**, 23
prospectives 131
prune belly syndrome 124
psychic alterations 95

renal failure malformations 95
retardation
  mental 94
  somatic 94
retractile testis 93

seminoma 87
  risk analysis, incidence 88
Sertoli cells 36, **37**
  fetal 15, **16**, 35
  function 64
  histometry 67
  Sa-type 35, **37**, **46**, 50
  Sb-type 35, **37**, **46**, 50
  Sc-type 35, **37**, **42**, **46**
  single cell volume 36
sperm analysis 72
spermatocytes 35, **40**
spermatogonia, A-type 35
  B-type 35, **39**
spermatogonia count 47
staged orchiopexy 120
  results **117**
standard orchiopexy 117
syndromes **94**

teratocarcinoma 87
testicular atrophy causes 86, 120
  anoxia 87
  chemical toxin 87
  histotoxin 87
  torsion 87
testicular cancer 83
testicular descent, embryology 11
  evolution 6
  in man **18**, **23**
  in mouse **24**
  in rodents 23
testicular fixation, different methods 115
testicular steroids, biosynthesis **61**
testicular tumor 128
  incidence **89**

risk 84
  5-year survival rate 89
testicular volume **98**
testis 12
  coverings 21
  differentiation 12
  morphometric analysis 36
  preoperative localization 115
  puberty 35
  torsion 95
testosterone, pathways 61, 62
testosterone secretion, in cryptorchid boys 65, 66
transfemoral arteriography 116
transient spermatogonium **14**, **49**
treatment schedule 128

tumor cell types 87
two-hit theory 91

ultrasonography 116
unilateral orchitis, experimental 76
unilateral testicular agenesis 29

Wolffian duct 17, 23, 64
  peristaltic 25

zinc 86

Urology in Childhood

By D. I. Williams; T. M. Barratt; H. B. Eckstein; S. M. Kohlinsky,
G. H. Newns; P. E. Polani; J. D. Singer.

1974. 280 figures. XXIII, 458 pages.
(Handbuch der Urologie, Suppl. 15)
ISBN 3-540-06406-0

Diagnostic Imaging of the Kidney and Urinary Tract in Children

By A. R. Chrispin, I. Gordon, C. Hall, C. Metreweli

1980. 271 figures in 418 separate illustrations. XVIII, 206 pages
(Current Diagnostic Pediatrics)
ISBN 3-540-09472-5

”...an eagerly awaited and good book. We would all like to learn
Great Ormond Street standards for looking after sick children. I
have also looked forward to GOS teaching on integrating radiographic, ultrasound and nuclear medicine studies. The book
copes with these high expectations...Persuade your library to
buy it even if you cannot.” *Clinical Radiology*

A. T. K. Cockett, K. Koshiba

Manual of Urologic Surgery

Illustrated by I. Takamoto

1979. 532 color illustrations. XVIII, 284 pages
(Comprehensive Manuals of Surcigal Specialties)
ISBN 3-540-90423-9

”This is a fine manual for students as well as practising urolo-
gist.As the authors mention, the illustrations demonstrate more
clearly than ordinary colour photographs many of the important
steps in everyday urological precedures... The illustrations are so
superb that the accompanying commentary is almost super-
fluous, although very clear and concise an absolute must for any
institution or individual who is concerned with the practice and
teaching of urology.” *South African Medical Journal*

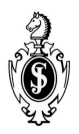
Springer-Verlag
Berlin
Heidelberg
New York

Clinical Practice in Urology

Series Editor:
Chisolm, G. D.

Urinary Diversion

Edited by **Michael Handley Ashken,** BSc, MS, FRCS
Consultant Urologist, Norfolk and Norwich Hospital, Norwich
1982. 53 figures. 168 pages ISBN 3-540-11273-1

Contents: Urinary Diversion in Neuro-Vesical Dysfunction.–
Urinary Diversion in Children.– Ureterosigmoidostomy in Chil-
dren.– Urinary Diversion in Malignant Disease.– Stoma Care.–
Urinary Reservoirs.– Subject Index.

The decision to create a urinary diversion ranks among one of
the most important in urological practice, Yet despite the far-
reaching consequences of this decision for the patient, urologists
often confine themselves to a single operative technique which,
though reliable, is not always the optimal solution to the
problem at hand.

Urinary Diversion is a presentation of proven alternatives to the
"one operation" approach. In it, leading urologic specialists
discuss the wide range of both conservative and operative procedures currently available for tailoring to an individual patient's
needs. The result of considerable personal experience with the
methods covered, the book highlights:

- the conservative management of neurovesical dysfunction,
  including urodynamic assessment, intermittent self-cathete-
  rization, and drug therapy

- urinary diversion in children with congenital and neurovesical
  disorders

- uroterosygmoidostomy in children, with emphasis on the
  importance and methods of long-term surveillance

- the effect of socio-economic and environmental factors in the
  choice of urinary diversion

- the role of the stomatherapist, including an up-to-date, practical guide to appliances and stoma care, and

- a critical appraisal of urinary reservoirs and appliance-free
  urinary diversion.

Carefully edited to avoid unnecessay repetition, *Urinary
Diversion* is an indispensable addition to the working library of
every urologist.

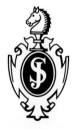

Springer-Verlag
Berlin
Heidelberg
New York